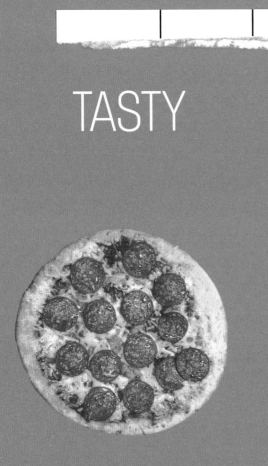

TASTY

STILL
TASTY

940 kcals

450 kcals

STILL TASTY

STILL **TASTY**

**Reduced-calorie versions
of 100 absolute favourite meals**

Graeme Tomlinson

EBURY
PRESS

CONTENTS

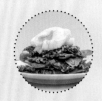

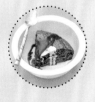

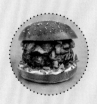

How your body weight is defined

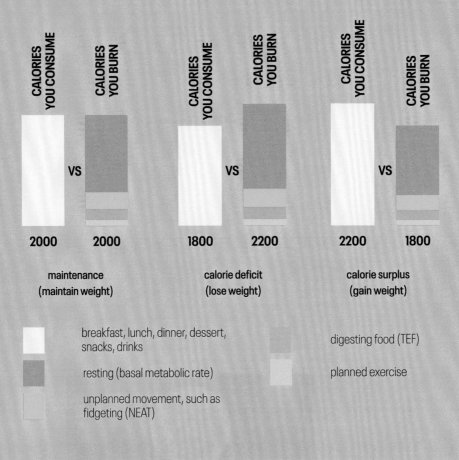

CALORIES YOU CONSUME | VS | CALORIES YOU BURN

2000 / 2000 — maintenance (maintain weight)

1800 / 2200 — calorie deficit (lose weight)

2200 / 1800 — calorie surplus (gain weight)

breakfast, lunch, dinner, dessert, snacks, drinks

resting (basal metabolic rate)

unplanned movement, such as fidgeting (NEAT)

digesting food (TEF)

planned exercise

INTRODUCTION

You can eat all the tasty recipes you love AND lose weight.

Yep, you can eat all your favourite foods. You won't find pizza, pasta, potatoes, bread, sugar and cream in many weight-loss cookbooks, but they're here. Why? Because there's no need to cut them out of your diet.

No single food makes you lose or gain weight.

The only scientifically proven principle to losing weight is to consume **fewer calories than you burn to create a calorie deficit.**

Despite all the weight-loss methods and strategies you've heard over the years, none will work unless you achieve a calorie deficit.

A lot of weight-loss advice is confusing – forbidding so-called 'bad' foods that supposedly make you gain weight, for example, such as cake or chocolate, or championing foods such as avocados as being 'good' for you.

While some foods are more nutritious than others, they all contain a calorie value.

You can eat pizza, burgers, lasagne, spaghetti carbonara, toasted sandwiches, pancakes with streaky bacon, cheesecake and sticky toffee pudding, for example, and lose weight if you remain within your calorie deficit.

Because they are usually higher in calories, if you eat them often you will find it harder to stay within a calorie deficit.

So, you have two options:

1. Only eat your favourite calorie-dense dishes now and then and make adjustments to your diet around enjoying them, so they don't negatively impact on your calorie deficit.
2. Keep eating all your favourite recipes, but reduce the calories they contain, so that you enjoy them regularly AND lose weight.

I'm here to help you with option 2.

Weight loss is not an experiment

It does not happen because you eat certain foods and exclude others, or eat at certain times of the day, or choose to eat smaller meals regularly as opposed to larger meals less frequently. It occurs when you find a sustainable, enjoyable, convenient way to maintain a calorie deficit over a period of time. That's it.

In my first book, *Eat What You Like & Lose Weight for Life*, I dispel many food myths, empowering you to understand that you can eat any food you like.

In this new book, you will find 100 reduced-calorie versions of some of your favourite breakfasts, lunches, dinners and desserts, as voted for by my Instagram followers around the world.

All recipes use easily available ingredients and give you the calorie and macronutrient information you need. But perhaps most importantly, they show you how you can easily reduce the calories in your favourite dishes while still enjoying the same amount of tasty food.

The calorie values of the 'tasty' versions of these recipes have been taken from popular recipe pages and brands around the world. Note that the 'tasty' calorie values of some dishes may change slightly depending on what your favourite version or brand of your favourite food is. I've included these to show you how many calories you can save with simple changes.

I've focused on keeping the delicious taste of the original dish and have used most of the same ingredients, to make the same volume of food on your plate (I am not interested in small portions and feeling hungry after a meal), but I've significantly reduced the calories in each one.

Most recipes are based on a single portion apart from where otherwise stated – where it is more practical to make a larger dish, such as a pie or pasta bake. But feel free to multiply or divide the ingredients to cater for a crowd or to reduce portion sizes to suit your meal preparations.

I wrote this book to show you that, despite popular dieting trends suggesting otherwise, the longevity of your weight-loss success ultimately comes down to how much you enjoy the method of calorie deficit you choose.

You want a diet of foods that you enjoy eating and get the body changes you desire long-term. This means you need to be aware of, and in control of, all calories you eat and drink, but more crucially, not restrict your diet.

You can opt for diets that omit certain food groups, such as keto, paleo and slimming clubs, if you like. And you can restrict your eating to certain times, with intermittent fasting, for example, if that helps you stick within a calorie deficit.

But you have to be honest and ask yourself: do I enjoy this? Do I know why this method works for me? Can I follow this method for the rest of my life? If the answer is no, then stop doing it.

Instead of looking for another new diet, which turns your life upside down, makes it hard to socialize with friends or eat as a family, focus on achieving your fat-loss goals by making small adjustments to your existing diet.

These small changes are the route to long-term weight-loss success. Start by finding your favourite meals in this book, and get cooking.

I am not a trained chef, I am a man who loves cooking and eating tasty food and wants as many people as possible to understand the simple basics of nutrition. These recipes were all tested and retested by me, in my normal kitchen at home, with regular pans, not many utensils and a standard oven. They are simple to prepare and they make modifying your daily diet as easy as possible for you.

Understanding what makes a balanced diet

There are three things that make up a supportive and balanced diet and I've considered all of these with the recipes in this book.

Energy balance – which decides your body mass. The average calories of the food and drink you consume must be lower than the amount of calories you burn through movement if you want to lose weight.

Nutrients – eat and drink a wide variety of foods that give you a variety of vitamins and minerals that your body needs to function.

Enjoyment – the enjoyment you get from food contributes to your happiness, a delicate component of your mental health.

All three are equally important.

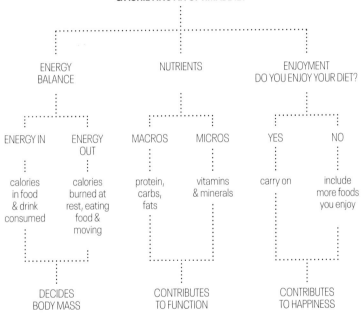

THE 3 PILLARS TO UNDERSTANDING & ACHIEVING AN OPTIMAL DIET

ENERGY BALANCE — NUTRIENTS — ENJOYMENT DO YOU ENJOY YOUR DIET?

ENERGY IN — ENERGY OUT — MACROS — MICROS — YES — NO

calories in food & drink consumed — calories burned at rest, eating food & moving — protein, carbs, fats — vitamins & minerals — carry on — include more foods you enjoy

DECIDES BODY MASS — CONTRIBUTES TO FUNCTION — CONTRIBUTES TO HAPPINESS

For decades we have been told that we need to follow diets which severely restrict the amount of food we eat, exclude specific foods or conform to rigid meal plans if we want to achieve our goals. All of which are often expensive and involve sacrifice, can be confusing and encourage you to have a negative relationship with food based on guilt, and are unsustainable.

There's no need to replace the food you love with food you don't. Understanding portion sizes and making small changes to your favourite foods to achieve a calorie deficit is not only more enjoyable, but much easier.

Small changes, big results

Here are a couple of examples of very small, simple adjustments to ingredients which have no impact on the enjoyment of your food, but crucially have a big impact on your calorie deficit over time.

Measure the oil you use to cook, let's say, your steak. What does it weigh? For example, 20ml of olive oil is 180 calories – 180 calories of your meal will be made up from oil alone. By reducing this to 5ml, you immediately cut 135 calories from your meal. You may want to reduce calories even further by using spray oil instead.

COOKING DINNER

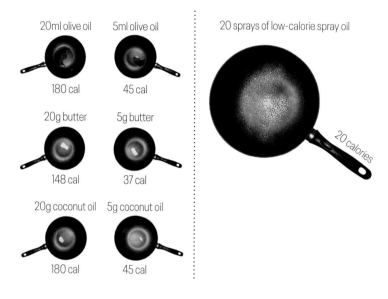

20ml olive oil   5ml olive oil   20 sprays of low-calorie spray oil

180 cal   45 cal

20g butter   5g butter

148 cal   37 cal

20g coconut oil   5g coconut oil

180 cal   45 cal

20 calories

You still enjoy the delicious steak and the taste and texture of cooking with the oil, but for significantly fewer calories.

Another example – you can still enjoy a cheese sandwich, filled with 100g Cheddar cheese (416 calories). Swapping full-fat Cheddar for the same amount of a 50% reduced-fat Cheddar (244 calories) allows you to eat the same amount of cheese in your sandwich but save 172 calories from the cheese alone. How you start the sandwich makes a huge difference too...

As you will see from my recipes, these opportunities are everywhere – you just need to appreciate they exist. Losing weight is as much about your ability to maintain and sustain behaviour change as it is about achieving a calorie deficit, so making these changes as easy as possible is a no-brainer.

Psychologically, weight loss can be seen as a series of easy adjustments to the food you already enjoy, made over time.

THE BEGINNING
OF A SANDWICH

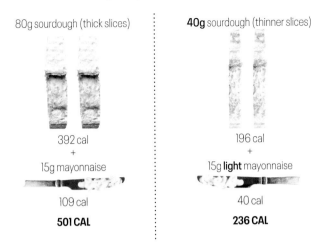

80g sourdough (thick slices)

392 cal
+
15g mayonnaise

109 cal

501 CAL

40g sourdough (thinner slices)

196 cal
+
15g **light** mayonnaise

40 cal

236 CAL

In some cases, one small tweak to a recipe can save hundreds of calories. In other cases, the accumulation of a few easy swaps brings about the same calorie savings to help achieve your calorie deficit while enabling you to enjoy filling portions of your favourite dishes.

JUST EATING
'healthyish' food to lose weight

'some pasta'
(120g)

'some cheddar'
(100g)

'some veggies/
seasoning'

'some pesto'
(60g)

1201 cal

INFORMED EATING
that supports my goal: 500–550 cal meal

75g pasta
supports my goal

50g low-fat cheddar
to support my goal

very low calories so I
don't need to weigh
them

40g low-fat pesto to
support my goal

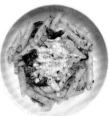

526 cal

Swaps that resemble the food you love

Unlike many reduced-calorie recipes designed for weight loss, you won't find any substitutes that bear no resemblance to the original food you enjoy here. No 'courgetti spaghetti' instead of spaghetti. No 'cauli rice', just rice. Ordinary bread and potatoes. No 'healthy' sugar substitutes that end up providing the same amount of calories, just simple sugar.

The reason you want bread is because you enjoy bread. It doesn't make sense to swap this with something that doesn't taste like or resemble the bread you love. There are some foods that offer lower calorie alternatives that taste very similar. These are easy opportunities to reduce your calorie intake whilst eating the same amount without sacrificing the tastes you enjoy.

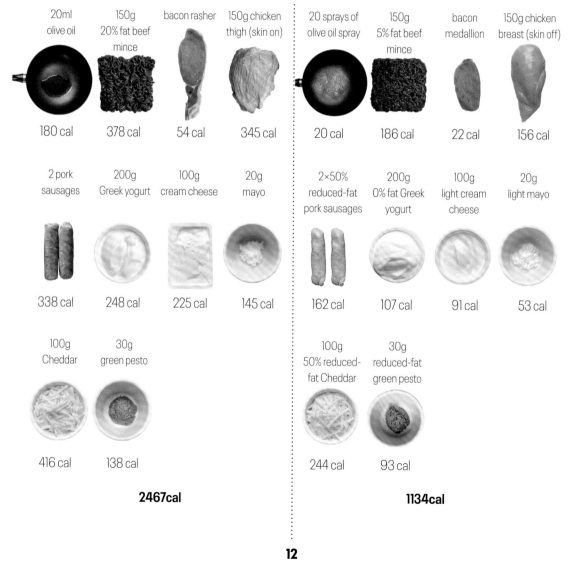

20ml olive oil	150g 20% fat beef mince	bacon rasher	150g chicken thigh (skin on)	20 sprays of olive oil spray	150g 5% fat beef mince	bacon medallion	150g chicken breast (skin off)
180 cal	378 cal	54 cal	345 cal	20 cal	186 cal	22 cal	156 cal
2 pork sausages	200g Greek yogurt	100g cream cheese	20g mayo	2×50% reduced-fat pork sausages	200g 0% fat Greek yogurt	100g light cream cheese	20g light mayo
338 cal	248 cal	225 cal	145 cal	162 cal	107 cal	91 cal	53 cal
100g Cheddar	30g green pesto			100g 50% reduced-fat Cheddar	30g reduced-fat green pesto		
416 cal	138 cal			244 cal	93 cal		

2467cal   **1134cal**

Understanding portion sizes

No single food can influence your diet for good or bad. A food can be high in calories, but if you eat a small portion then it can still support your weight-loss goal. Similarly, a food can be low in calories, but if you eat too much of it then it will no longer help you achieve your calorie deficit (and you won't have a balanced diet that comes from eating a variety of foods).

A food can be high in many micronutrients, meaning you only need to eat a small portion to obtain its many vitamins and minerals. If you eat lots of some micronutrient-dense foods, like nuts, they also contain a high number of calories, so will make eating within a calorie deficit hard.

If you eat a lot of food that is low in micronutrients, like chips or crisps, you'd have to eat lots of it to get the vitamins and minerals you need and along with that you'd be eating a lot of calories too.

The easiest way to understand the portion sizes of the food you eat is to weigh it.

All you need is an inexpensive set of kitchen scales. This enables you to accurately align the quantity of food you eat with your individual calorie requirements.

Are you in a calorie deficit?

THE FAT LOSS CHECKLIST
are you in a calorie deficit?

YES · · · · · · · · · · · NO · · · · · · · · · · · DON'T KNOW

Do you enjoy it? · · · · ·

Move more · · · · Reduce calories · · · · Track calories & understand your requirements

YES · · · · NO

Carry on · · · · Find a more enjoyable method

You can get your calorie target for your specific goal for free by visiting www.fitnesschef.uk and following the simple steps.

In time, you may become familiar with what particular portion sizes look like. But until then, the scales show you how many calories you are eating.

The ingredients in these recipes have quantities listed, so you just need to weigh the ingredients when preparing them. If you think weighing food is time-consuming, just imagine it as your assistant that helps you combine the food you love with your calorie deficit.

Macronutrients and calorie reduction

You'll notice that many of my still tasty recipes are lower in fat than the original version. This doesn't mean that fat is 'bad', it is simply because it is the most calorie-dense macronutrient.

Reducing it is the easiest way to cut calories while maintaining portion sizes. But remember, it's overall calories that are important for losing, maintaining or gaining weight, and there is a place for all three macronutrients (fat, carbs and protein) in different quantities depending on your personal preferences.

You may ask, 'aren't reduced-fat alternatives bad because they replace the fat with sugar?' Well, no.

Firstly, because no food, sugar included, is inherently bad.

Secondly, because reduced-calorie foods offer you the perfect opportunity to eat the same amount of a food that's very similar to one you enjoy, but for fewer calories, which supports your calorie deficit.

A word on protein

Most of these recipes are relatively high in protein. This is because a diet high in protein is more likely to make you feel full, making you less likely to overeat.

Protein also has a higher thermic effect than carbs and fats, meaning that, over time, protein burns significantly more calories than fats and carbs during digestion. Over a long period of time this is significant.

I recommend consistently aiming for 1–2g protein per kg of bodyweight a day. You can find out more, for free, about your daily protein goals, if you'd like to know more, on my website.

Everything in moderation – but how do you measure moderation?

The old adage about eating a balanced diet with 'everything in moderation' is very true. But a balanced diet can only be measured with your knowledge and judgement. Know the caloric requirements for your weight-loss goal, understand which foods are nutritious for your body, and develop consistent judgement about how much of them you eat.

Unlike counting calories, it is extremely difficult to calculate the micronutrients you eat, and nutrient-dense foods usually contain a vast array. To attempt to count these would be exhausting.

My advice is to try to source your nutrients from whole foods such as meat, fish and vegetables in main dishes rather than snacks because meals offer larger quantities of different foods, enabling you to eat higher amounts of a variety of nutrients. This also leaves snacks as opportunities to enjoy smaller portions of less nutritious, possibly calorie-dense, foods you love.

Your sweet spot is the middle ground

The first step to making your relationship with food as good as possible is to equip yourself with simple facts. No individual food or food group can derail your goal. But guilt, shame and misinformation about the food you eat can. It can propel you on to a dieting roundabout where you can't succeed, but you can't get off either. Get into bed with the food facts, not the people in the fitness industry who just want your money.

The most important thing is not knowing which foods to avoid, but how to make sure you can include any food you enjoy in your diet. This is why knowing more about the food you eat instead of giving it a moral power over you is much more useful. You can then always adapt and be flexible to help yourself stay on track to achieve your weight-loss goal. Even if you overeat today, there is always tomorrow.

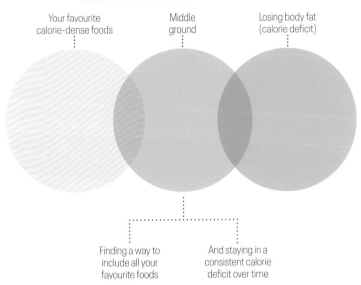

ENJOYING YOUR DIET & ACHIEVING YOUR GOALS

Your favourite calorie-dense foods

Middle ground

Losing body fat (calorie deficit)

Finding a way to include all your favourite foods

And staying in a consistent calorie deficit over time

The second step is to ignore anyone, including professionals, who tell you that you should never eat a particular food. Unless you have a medical condition, such advice comes without any context about what you need or enjoy.

A slice of cheesecake isn't a particularly nutritious choice because it doesn't contain many micronutrients, but out of a week of 21 meals and 14–16 snacks, the slice of cheesecake is fairly insignificant. Flexibility and inclusion brings enjoyment. Extremism, rigidity and exclusion can bring about a toxic, warped relationship with the food you eat. Choose the former.

Tactical snacking

Snacking has been an area of much confusion over the years. Many have been told they must eat nutritious snacks to support their weight-loss goal and exclude favourites such as chocolate or crisps.

But as no food is good or bad when it comes to weight loss, it's the quantity and the calories it contains that is the key.

Even so-called 'good' nutrient-dense foods such as nuts or avocado are calorie dense.

If you're looking to optimize your calorie intake, nutrient consumption and enjoyment to form an optimal diet, snack times may be the perfect opportunity to include much-loved, less nutritious foods within your calorie needs, providing you're getting enough nutrients from your main meals.

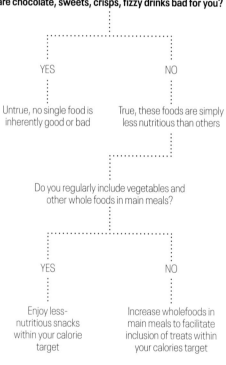

BALANCING NUTRIENTS & ENJOYMENT
are chocolate, sweets, crisps, fizzy drinks bad for you?

YES   NO

Untrue, no single food is inherently good or bad   True, these foods are simply less nutritious than others

Do you regularly include vegetables and other whole foods in main meals?

YES   NO

Enjoy less-nutritious snacks within your calorie target   Increase wholefoods in main meals to facilitate inclusion of treats within your calories target

Powerful patience

The dieting industry tells you that you need to make extreme changes to lose weight, but actually what you should to do to manage your weight for the rest of your life is very simple and not too far from what you are doing already.

Though small, informed adjustments to the ingredients you already eat might not be as sexy as a 'miracle 4-week fat-loss diet', these tweaks add up to make a huge difference over time.

Instead of a diet that yo-yos up and down because you hate yourself and take drastic action, only to eventually regain all the weight you lose, you can love yourself, become informed and take slow, steady, enjoyable action that lasts a lifetime.

Slower fat loss ends up being faster than rapid fat loss simply because rapid fat loss is unsustainable over time.

WHY SLOWER FAT LOSS IS FASTER

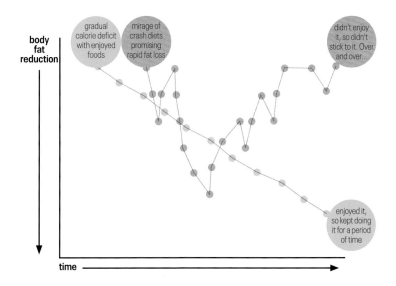

No more pressure

Unlike many weight-loss cookbooks, I give you permission to eat any food you like – I want to remove any pressure from you. You don't have to follow a specific meal plan to achieve your goals. You don't have to exclude any food groups or prepare complicated recipes with countless ingredients. All you have to do is enjoy achieving a calorie deficit – that's the only way you'll stick to it.

Let this book be a lifelong source of tasty, lower-calorie meals, allowing you to enjoy many of your favourite recipes, day in day out. I hope it empowers you with the confidence that losing weight can be as simple as making a few very small changes to your life. Most of all, I hope it assures you that you can lose weight and keep it off by enjoying your favourite foods.

Your weight does not define who you are, nor does it define your worth. But if you believe that losing or maintaining your weight will improve your happiness, I truly hope this book serves as a valuable resource in your life to make it more enjoyable for you.

Best wishes!

Now, let's make some food!

Graeme

BREAKFASTS

The science says that eating or skipping breakfast has no effect on whether you lose or gain weight. What may be important is *what* you eat for breakfast, as well as managing your overall calorie intake to achieve a calorie deficit over a period of time.

Evidence aside, technically you never skip breakfast. Breakfast is simply the first meal you eat on any given day. You don't need to consume it at a specific time. If you prefer to eat as soon as you wake up, you can. If you prefer to eat your first meal of the day a little later, then do so. Do what suits you.

We are all different, there is no right or wrong here. If skipping an early meal means you overeat at other times during the day, then enjoying a calorie-controlled breakfast may be the best idea for you.

But if you aren't hungry first thing in the morning, then pushing back your first meal of the day by a few hours could be an easy way to support your calorie deficit for fat loss. Either way, I've got 15 delicious breakfast recipes for whenever you want to eat them.

I've highlighted the adjustments made to reduce the calories in each dish, but ensured that the main, delicious ingredients you love are not substituted with bland alternatives. These adjustments are small, but over weeks and months the reduction in calories could make a big difference to your weight loss. Enjoy!

BIG FRY-UP

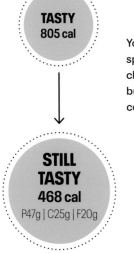

TASTY
805 cal

STILL TASTY
468 cal
P47g | C25g | F20g

You can still eat a fry-up and lose weight! Switch cooking oil for spray oil, bacon rashers for medallions and pork sausages for chicken sausages. You have to say goodbye to fried bread, sorry, but you still get toast and butter AND you reduce your calorie consumption by 337 calories.

TAKES 15 minutes

10 × sprays olive oil cooking spray
2 chicken sausages
3 bacon medallions
1 medium egg
½ tomato

Small handful of spinach
1 × 40g slice of white or
   wholemeal bread
5g unsalted butter
Salt and pepper

1. Spray a large frying pan with the oil and set over a medium heat. Add the chicken sausages and cook for 5 minutes.
2. Then add the bacon medallions and cook for a further 5 minutes until both the bacon and sausages are cooked through.
3. Reduce the heat slightly, then crack in the egg and add the tomato and spinach. Cook for 3–5 minutes until the yolk is cooked to your liking.
4. Toast the bread and serve buttered with your fry-up. Season with salt and pepper to your taste. Enjoy!

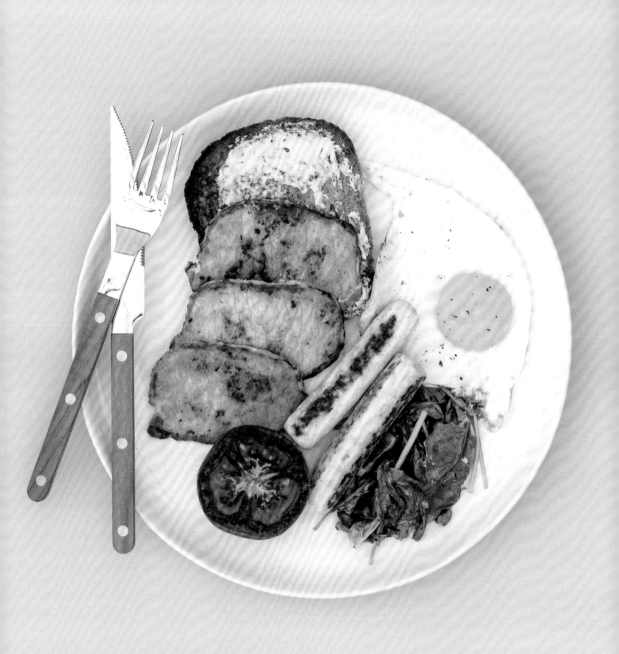

VEGETARIAN FRY-UP

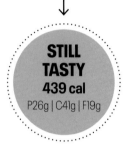

TASTY
574 cal

STILL
TASTY
439 cal
P26g | C41g | F19g

Just because your fry-up contains nutritious ingredients it doesn't mean that it supports your calorie deficit. By reducing the typical 20ml cooking oil to 5ml, you can still cook your fry-up perfectly while saving 135 calories – and enjoy exactly the same delicious taste!

TAKES 15 minutes

5ml olive oil
50g button mushrooms, roughly chopped
1 medium egg
1 tomato, halved
Small handful of freshly chopped flat-leaf parsley

30g halloumi cheese, thinly sliced
150g baked beans
1 × 40g slice of white or wholemeal bread
Salt and pepper

1. Put a frying pan over a medium heat. Add the olive oil and mushrooms and cook for 5 minutes until the mushrooms begin to shrink.
2. Make space in the pan, then crack in the egg and add the tomato, parsley and halloumi slices. Cook the egg for 3–5 minutes and the halloumi and tomato for 2 minutes on each side until browned.
3. While the fry-up is cooking, heat the baked beans in a small saucepan for 3 minutes until they begin to bubble. Toast the bread to your liking.
4. Transfer the contents of the frying pan to a serving plate, add the baked beans and toast, season with salt and pepper and serve.

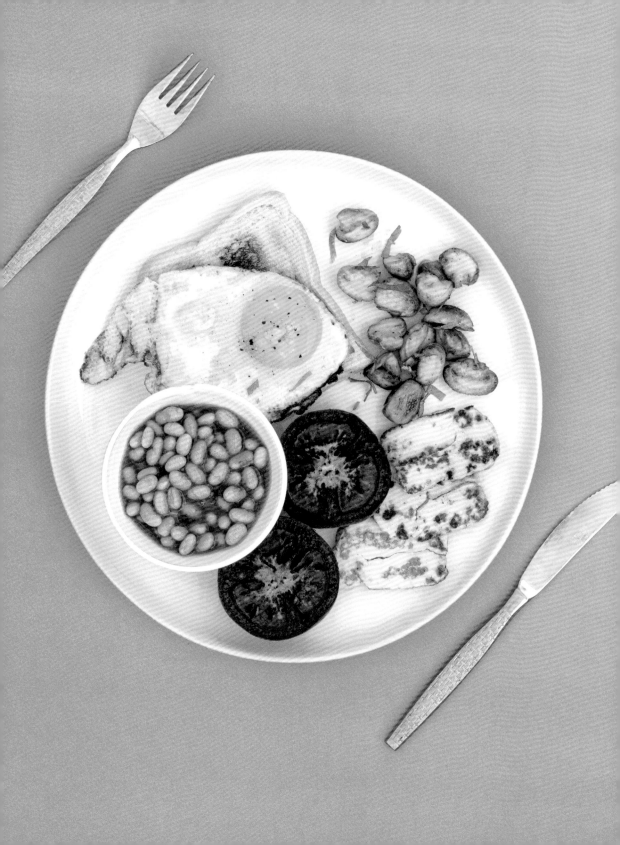

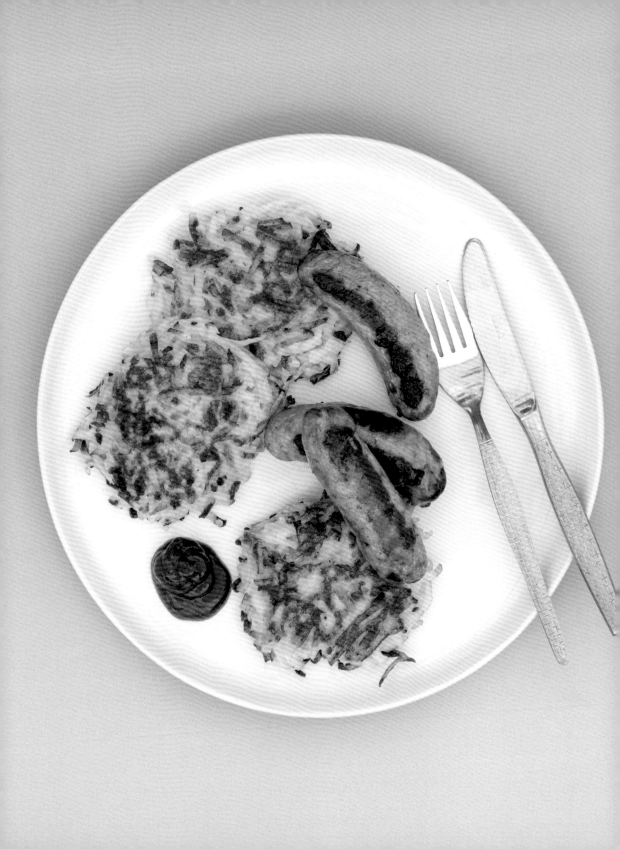

SAUSAGES & HASH BROWNS

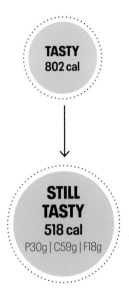

TASTY
802 cal

STILL TASTY
518 cal
P30g | C59g | F18g

Two of your favourite fry-up ingredients, but in greater quantities – what's not to love? By using reduced-fat pork sausages, switching 30ml olive oil for 30 sprays of oil and reducing the usual 10ml oil for preparing the hash browns to 2ml, you can save 284 calories and still enjoy a bumper breakfast!

TAKES 30 minutes

3 reduced-fat pork sausages
200g potatoes, peeled
¼ onion, finely chopped
20g plain flour

2ml olive oil
30 × sprays olive oil cooking spray
15g tomato ketchup
Salt

1. Preheat the oven to 200°C and place the sausages on a foil-lined tray. Cook for 25–30 minutes, turning halfway through cooking.
2. While the sausages are cooking, grate the potatoes into a large bowl using a cheese grater.
3. Clench the grated potatoes in your hands and squeeze out as much water as possible before returning to the bowl. You may need to repeat this 2–3 times.
4. Add the onion, flour, olive oil and a pinch of salt to the potatoes and toss thoroughly with your hands to combine.
5. Spray a frying pan with the oil and put over a medium heat.
6. Make 3 hash brown patties with your hands, adding them to the pan at the same time. Cook for 3–4 minutes on each side or until golden brown and crispy.
7. Serve the sausages with the hash browns, adding ketchup on the side.

RED PEPPER HASH BROWN STACK
with poached eggs

Here's another simple hash brown recipe, but this time with added eggs. Still tasty and 360 calories less than the original.

READY IN 15 minutes

200g potatoes, peeled	20g plain flour
¼ onion, finely chopped	30 × sprays olive oil cooking spray
¼ red pepper, finely chopped	2 medium eggs
1 tsp paprika	Small handful of spinach
1 tsp mixed herbs	Salt and pepper

1. Grate the potatoes into a large bowl using a cheese grater.
2. Clench the grated potatoes in your hands and squeeze out as much water as possible before returning to the bowl. You may need to repeat this 2–3 times.
3. Add the onions, red pepper, paprika, mixed herbs, flour and a pinch of salt to the potatoes. Toss thoroughly with your hands to combine.
4. Spray a medium frying pan with the oil and set over a medium heat.
5. Make 3 hash brown patties with your hands, adding them to the pan at the same time. Cook for 3–4 minutes on each side or until golden brown and crispy.
6. Half-fill a deep frying pan or wok with water, bring to a simmer and delicately break the eggs into the water. Poach for 3–5 minutes until cooked to your liking, then remove with a slotted spoon and drain on a plate.
7. Stack up the hash browns with the spinach, top with the poached eggs with and season with salt and pepper if you wish.

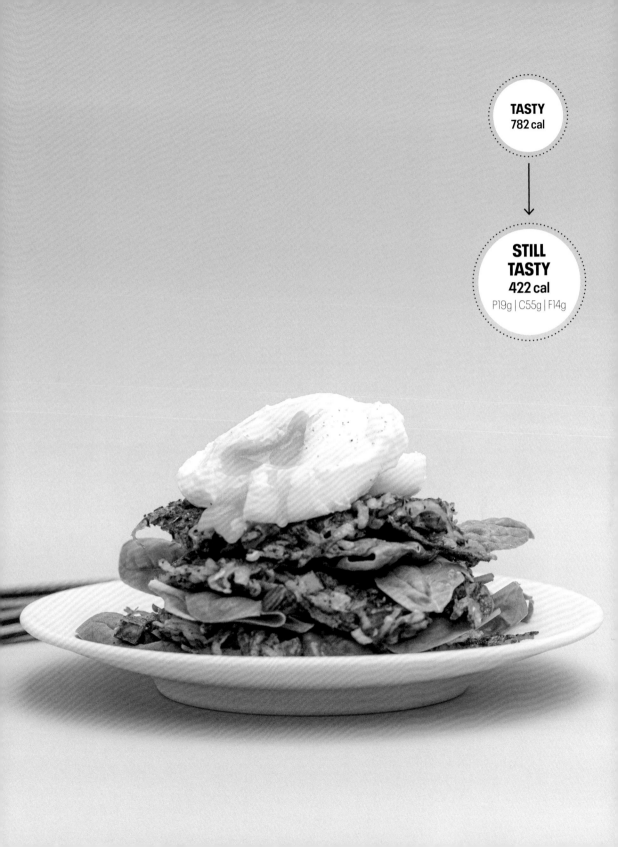

TASTY
782 cal

STILL
TASTY
422 cal
P19g | C55g | F14g

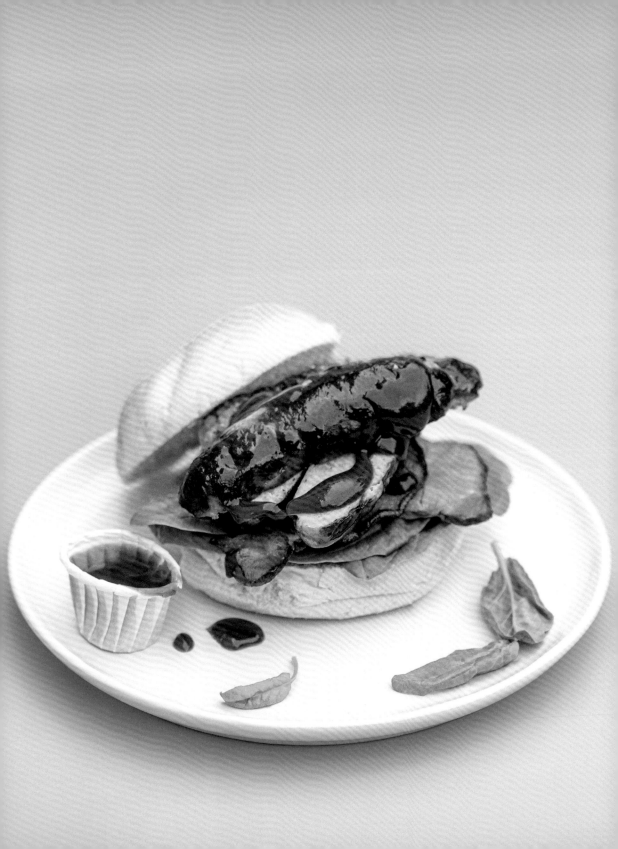

SAUSAGE & BACON
BREAKFAST ROLL

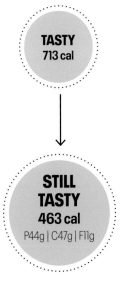

TASTY
713 cal

STILL TASTY
463 cal
P44g | C47g | F11g

High-street breakfast rolls are often full of calories, but if you make your own with bacon medallions instead of the rashers, leave out the butter and use reduced-fat pork sausages, you save 250 calories – and it tastes just as good!

TAKES 20 minutes

2 reduced-fat pork sausages
4 bacon medallions
60g white roll
Small handful of spinach

For the brown sauce
15g tomato purée
10ml water
¼ onion, finely chopped
5g brown sugar
10ml white wine vinegar
10ml Worcestershire sauce
Sprinkle of paprika
Sprinkle of salt and pepper

1. Preheat the grill to medium. Grill the sausages for 10 minutes.
2. Turn the sausages over, add the bacon medallions and grill for 10–12 minutes, turning the bacon medallions halfway through cooking.
3. While the sausages and bacon are cooking, put the brown sauce ingredients in a blender and blitz until smooth. Pour into a small saucepan and heat gently for 3–4 minutes. Keep stirring with a wooden spoon until the sauce thickens.
4. Split the white roll open and fill with the grilled sausages, bacon medallions, spinach and tangy brown sauce. Serve.

CHEESY SCRAMBLED EGGS
ON TOAST

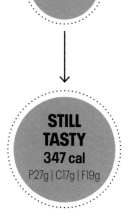

TASTY
457 cal

STILL TASTY
347 cal
P27g | C17g | F19g

Scrambled eggs still taste wonderful without cream and milk. Just use reduced-fat Cheddar cheese instead of the regular version to save 110 calories and enjoy a simple, delicious breakfast.

TAKES 10 minutes

3 medium eggs
20g reduced-fat Cheddar cheese, grated
Small handful of freshly chopped chives

1 × 40g slice of white or wholemeal bread
Salt and pepper

1. Crack the eggs into a small bowl and beat with a fork until smooth. Add the grated cheese and chives and season with salt and pepper.
2. Put a medium saucepan over a low heat, add the egg mixture and cook for 5–7 minutes, scraping the pan with a spatula to ensure all the egg and cheese mixture cooks and scrambles evenly.
3. Meanwhile, toast the bread.
4. Finally, top the toast with your cheesy eggs and season with more salt and pepper, if you like.

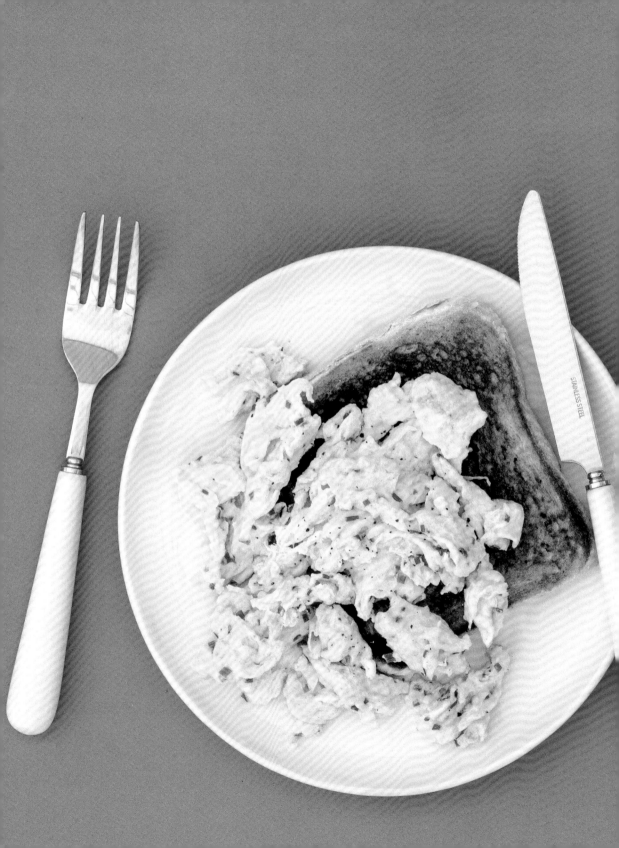

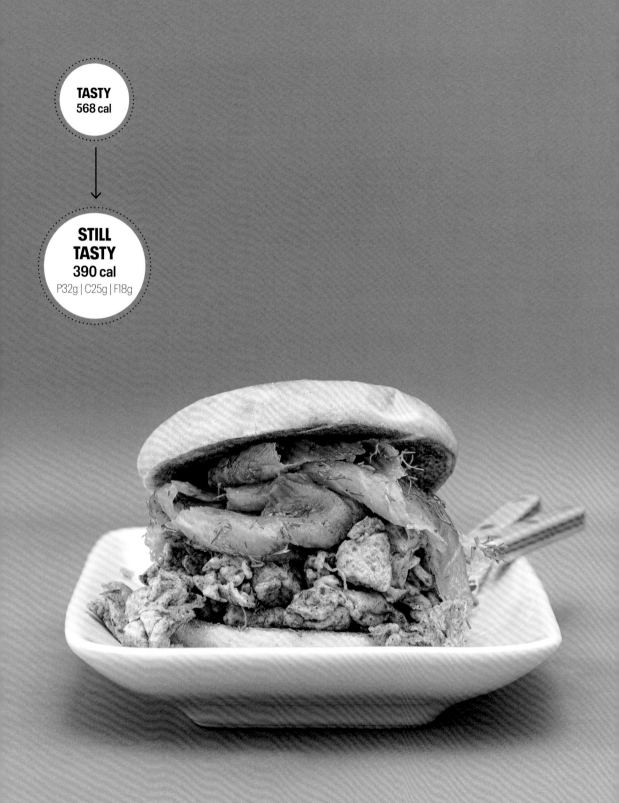

TASTY
568 cal

STILL
TASTY
390 cal
P32g | C25g | F18g

SCRAMBLED EGG
& DILL-INFUSED
SMOKED SALMON BAGEL

Scrambled eggs are back! But this time combining the classic flavours of smoked salmon and dill to give you a protein-rich breakfast oozing beneficial fats. Many people add butter to scrambled eggs, but they are equally delicious without it. In fact, by foregoing 10g butter and swapping your usual bagel for a tasty bagel thin, you can save 178 calories and still enjoy a nutritious, flavour-packed first meal of the day.

TAKES 10 minutes

2 medium eggs	1 tbsp freshly chopped dill
1 tsp paprika	1 bagel thin, halved
75g smoked salmon	Pepper

1. Crack the eggs into a small bowl, then add the paprika and a twist of black pepper. Whisk with a fork until smooth.
2. Put a medium pan over a low heat, add the egg mixture and cook for 5–7 minutes, scraping the pan with a spatula to ensure all the egg mixture cooks and scrambles evenly.
3. While the eggs are cooking, coat both sides of the smoked salmon in the dill.
4. Lightly toast the bagel thin halves.
5. Fill the toasted bagel thin with the scrambled eggs and dill-coated smoked salmon and serve.

EGGS BENEDICT

This worldwide favourite will always be a winner. The most calorie-dense part of this delicious breakfast is usually the hollandaise sauce. So, swap 50g crème fraîche for a half-fat version and reduce the usual 50g butter to 5g to enjoy this classic just as much, but with 391 fewer calories, supporting your calorie deficit for fat loss.

TAKES 15 minutes

2 medium eggs, plus 1 egg yolk	25g Parma ham (2 slices)
50g half-fat crème fraîche	Small handful of freshly
5g Dijon mustard	chopped chives
2g unsalted butter	Pepper
70g English muffin	

1. To make the hollandaise sauce, you need a medium heatproof bowl that fits over a small saucepan. Add the egg yolk, crème fraîche and mustard to the bowl and whisk together with a fork.
2. Pour 200ml water into a small saucepan, bring to a simmer, then place the bowl over the saucepan. Add the butter and stir for 7–8 minutes until the sauce thickens. Turn off the heat.
3. Half-fill a deep frying pan or wok with water, bring to a simmer and delicately break the eggs into the water. Poach for 3–5 minutes until cooked to your liking, then remove with a slotted spoon and drain on a plate.
4. Meanwhile, slice the muffin in half and lightly toast both halves. Add a Parma ham slice to each half.
5. Carefully top each muffin half with a poached egg before spooning hot hollandaise sauce over the top. Sprinkle with chives and season with black pepper to taste. Serve.

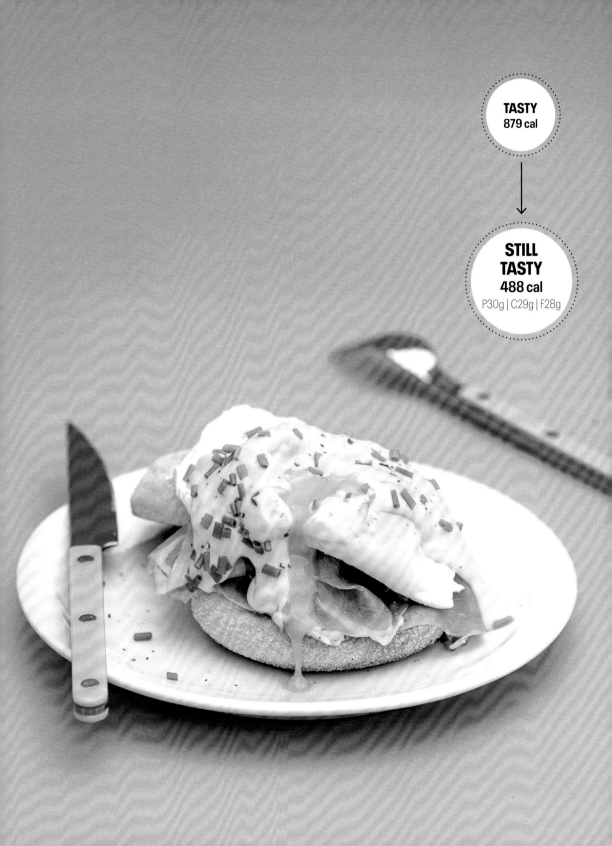

TASTY
879 cal

STILL
TASTY
488 cal
P30g | C29g | F28g

SERRANO HAM
& PARMESAN OMELETTE

By adding seasoning, vegetables and herbs to eggs, you can enjoy a great-tasting omelette and save calories to support your weight-loss goal. Here we are ditching the milk often added to eggs when whisking, adding seasoning and reducing the calorie-dense cooking oil from 20ml to 5ml and 20g Parmesan cheese to 10g. Great taste and an easy saving of 220 calories. Win-win.

TAKES 10 minutes

5ml olive oil
3 medium eggs
1 spring onion, finely chopped

10g shaved Parmesan
50g Serrano ham, sliced
Salt and pepper

1. Put a medium saucepan over a high heat and add the olive oil. Tilt the pan to spread the oil evenly over the base of the pan.
2. Crack the eggs into a small bowl, add the spring onion and season with salt and pepper. Whisk with a fork until smooth.
3. Add the egg mixture to the pan and allow to set for 20–30 seconds. Then manoeuvre the pan in a circular motion and lift up the cooked egg with a spatula to allow the uncooked egg underneath to cook. Repeat for 3–4 minutes until all of the egg mixture is nearly cooked.
4. Reduce the heat to low, add three-quarters of the Parmesan and Serrano ham to the centre of the omelette and fold the omelette in half with a spatula. Top with the remaining Parmesan and ham and cook for a further minute. Serve.

RED PEPPER, SPINACH,
TOMATO & MUSHROOM
OMELETTE

TASTY
455 cal

STILL TASTY
280 cal
P20g | C5g | F20g

This very easy veggie omelette swaps 20ml cooking oil for 5ml and loses the usual 50ml milk added to the eggs to make a delicious breakfast or brunch, packed full of micronutrients.

TAKES 10 minutes

5ml olive oil
3 medium eggs
4 cherry tomatoes, halved
3 button mushrooms, roughly chopped

¼ red pepper, roughly chopped
Small handful of spinach
Small handful of freshly chopped parsley
Salt and pepper

1. Put a medium saucepan over a high heat, add the oil and tilt the pan to spread the oil evenly over the base of the pan.
2. Crack the eggs into a small bowl and whisk with fork until smooth. Add the cherry tomatoes, mushrooms, red pepper, and spinach, season with salt and pepper and mix together with a fork.
3. Add the egg mixture to the pan and allow to set for 20–30 seconds. Then manoeuvre the pan in a circular motion and lift up the cooked egg with a spatula to allow the uncooked egg underneath to cook. Repeat for 3–4 minutes until all of the egg mixture is fully cooked.
4. Serve scattered with the parsley and more salt and pepper, if you like.

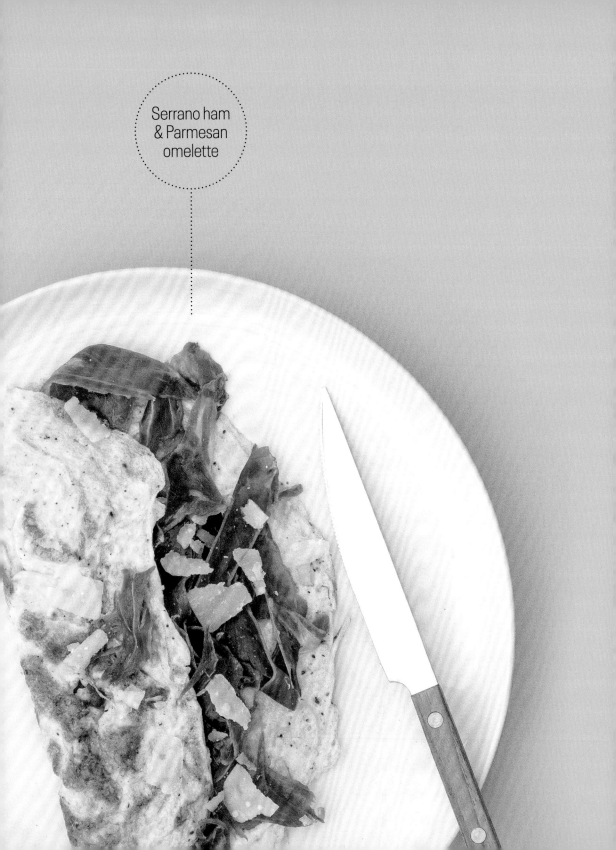

Serrano ham
& Parmesan
omelette

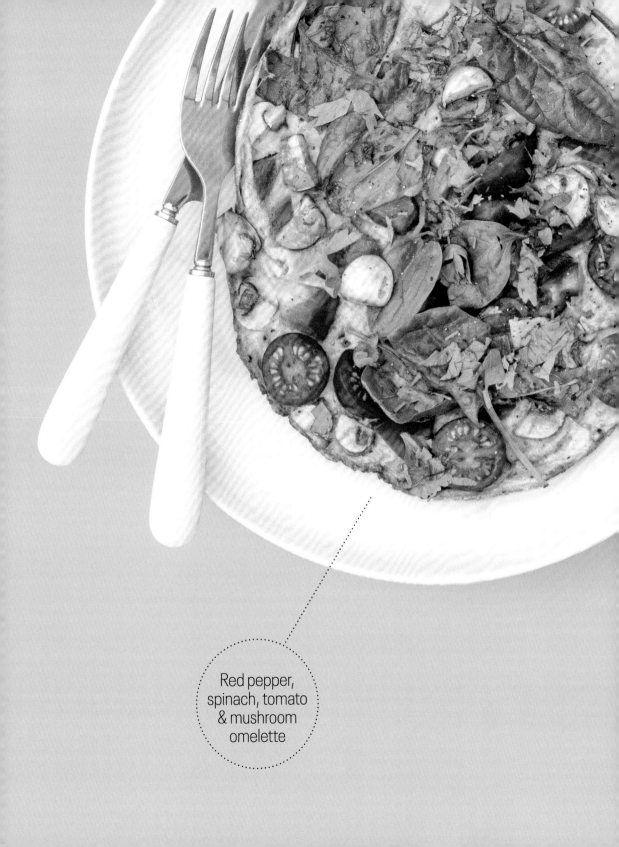

Red pepper, spinach, tomato & mushroom omelette

CRISPY BACON
& MAPLE SYRUP PANCAKES

Pancakes, bacon and maple syrup is a much-loved combination around the world. So, I didn't want to meddle with the heart and soul of this recipe, which means you'll still be enjoying streaky bacon and maple syrup! By adjusting the 15g butter to 5g, Greek yogurt to 0% fat Greek yogurt and reducing the 30ml maple syrup to 10ml, you get the fantastic taste of all your favourite ingredients AND save 133 calories.

READY IN 15 minutes
MAKES 4 pancakes

3 rashers of unsmoked streaky bacon
65g plain flour
1 tsp ground cinnamon
1 tsp baking powder
50ml semi-skimmed milk

1 medium egg
50g 0% fat Greek yogurt
5g unsalted butter
10ml maple syrup
3 medium strawberries, hulled and halved

1. Preheat the grill to high. Put the bacon rashers on a foil-lined baking tray and grill for 5–7 minutes on each side until as crispy and golden as you desire.
2. Put the flour, cinnamon, baking powder, milk, egg and yogurt in a large bowl and mix with a fork until you have a smooth batter.
3. Put a large frying pan over a high heat. When the pan is hot, add the butter and tilt the pan to spread the butter evenly over the base of the pan.

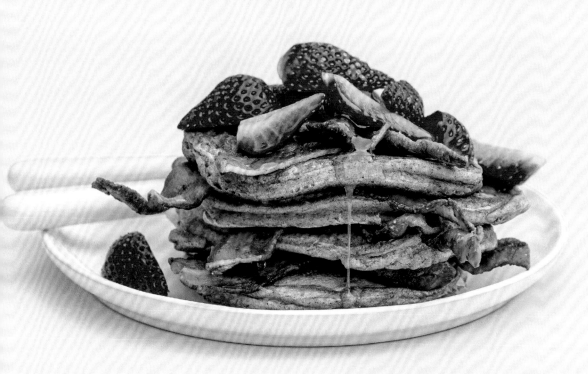

4. Spoon 2-tablespoon portions of batter into the pan. When the pancakes start to bubble, flip and cook for 30 seconds on the other side before plating. Repeat until you've used all the batter (you should have 4 pancakes in total).

5. Break the grilled streaky bacon into small strips. Then add to each layer of pancake as you stack them on top of each other. Drizzle the maple syrup over the top of the pancake stack.

6. Top with the strawberries and serve.

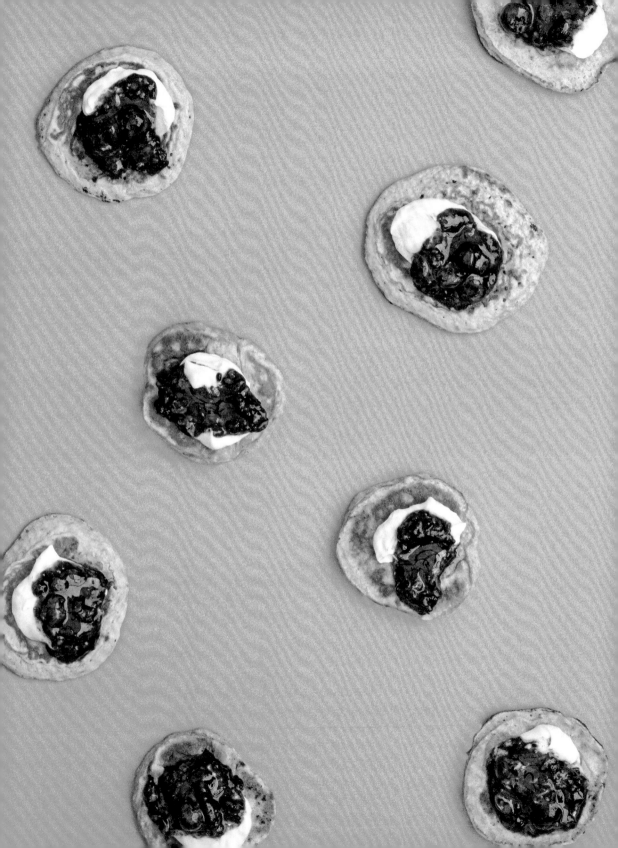

BERRY JAM PANCAKES

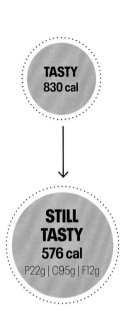

TASTY
830 cal

STILL TASTY
576 cal
P22g | C95g | F12g

Sweet ingredients definitely enhance the taste of pancakes, but you'd be surprised how easily you can pack the calories into the toppings you add. The great news is that you can reduce the calories but still maintain the sweetness with a delicious low-calorie jam made with minimal fuss. Simply swap a whole medium banana for half, 15g honey for 5g, 15g butter for 5g and 50g strawberry jam for 150g crushed berries. Enjoy!

READY IN 10 minutes
MAKES 4 pancakes

75g plain flour
1 tsp baking powder
50ml semi-skimmed milk
1 medium egg
1 twist of salt
½ medium banana, mashed

5g unsalted butter
50g blueberries
50g raspberries
50g blackberries
50g 0% fat Greek yogurt
5g honey

1. Put the flour, baking powder, milk, egg, salt and mashed banana in a large bowl and mix with a fork until you have a smooth batter.
2. Put a large frying pan over a high heat. When the pan is hot, add the butter and tilt the pan to spread the butter evenly.
3. Spoon 2-tablespoon portions of batter into the pan. When the pancakes start to bubble, flip and cook for 30 seconds on the other side before plating. Repeat until you've used all the batter (you should have 4 pancakes).
4. Once the pancakes are cooked, put the blueberries, raspberries and blackberries in 3 separate small bowls and mash with a fork until you have a jam-like purée for each.
5. Stack the pancakes, layering each with mashed blueberries, raspberries and blackberries.
6. Finally, add Greek yogurt on the side of the plate and drizzle the honey over the pancakes. Serve.

SWEET POTATO PANCAKES
with fried egg

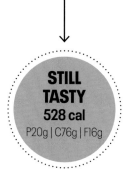

TASTY
609 cal

STILL TASTY
528 cal
P20g | C76g | F16g

By switching 5ml olive oil for 5 sprays of spray oil and reducing 10g butter to 5g, you can save 81 calories for this simple supper. It may not seem a lot, but over time these small savings add up to help you achieve your weight-loss goal. The best thing is that you can enjoy the same-sized portion and it still tastes delicious.

TAKES 15 minutes

250g sweet potatoes, peeled and chopped into 2cm cubes
30g plain flour
1 tsp baking powder
2 medium eggs
½ red onion, finely chopped

½ tsp salt
½ tsp black pepper
½ tsp dried Italian herbs
5g unsalted butter
5 × sprays butter flavour cooking spray

1. Half-fill a large saucepan with water, bring to the boil then add the chopped sweet potatoes. Simmer for 5–7 minutes until tender.
2. Drain the sweet potatoes and rinse in cold water to cool. Then transfer to a large bowl and mash with a potato masher until smooth. Add the flour, baking powder, 1 egg, the red onion, salt, black pepper and dried Italian herbs and mix thoroughly with your hands until evenly combined.
3. Set a large pan over a high heat and melt the butter. Spoon large tablespoons of the sweet potato mixture into the pan to make 4 × 1cm pancakes. Fry for 2–3 minutes on each side until slightly crispy. Then stack the pancakes on a serving plate.
4. Spray a separate small pan with the oil and set over a medium heat. Then crack in the remaining egg and fry for 3–4 minutes.
5. Top the pancake stack with the fried egg and serve with a garnish of coriander if you like.

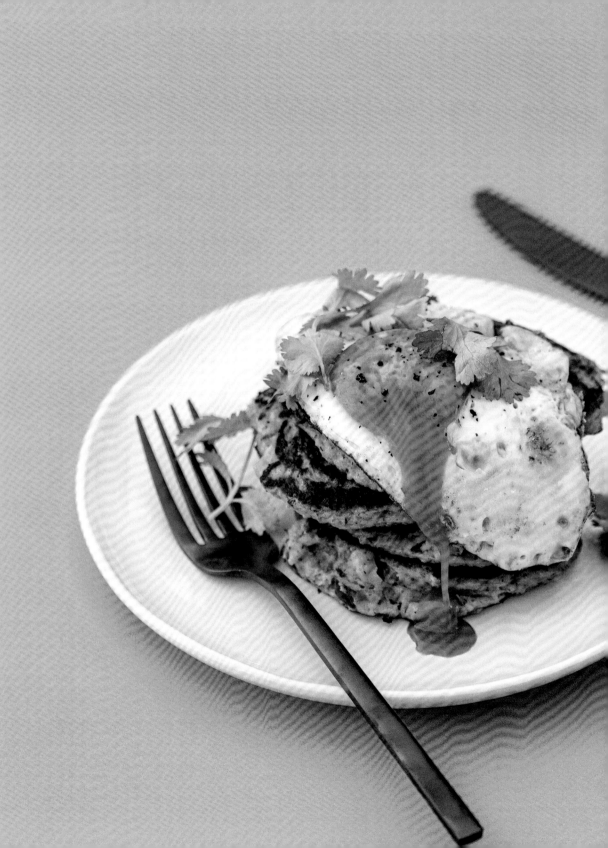

SHAKSHUKA

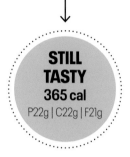

TASTY
455 cal

STILL TASTY
365 cal
P22g | C22g | F21g

This popular dish is already fairly low in calories, but by reducing the usual 15ml glug of olive oil to 5ml, you can enjoy exactly the same tasty meal, but save 90 calories. Across fifty shakshukas a year, that equals 4,500 calories without any sacrifice at all!

TAKES 20 minutes

5ml olive oil
1 onion, finely chopped
2 garlic cloves, crushed
1 red pepper, deseeded roughly chopped
100ml passata
Small handful of freshly chopped coriander

½ tsp ground cumin
Small handful of spinach, torn
3 vine tomatoes, finely chopped
3 medium eggs
Salt and pepper

1. Put a medium saucepan over a medium heat and add the olive oil, onion and garlic. Cook for 2 minutes until the onion begins to brown.
2. Add the red pepper, passata, coriander, cumin and spinach. Stir with a wooden spoon and cook for 2 minutes.
3. Then add the tomatoes, season with salt and pepper, stir and reduce the heat. Simmer, with a lid on, for 8–10 minutes until the sauce thickens.
4. Remove the lid, stir, then make 3 small indents with a wooden spoon. Crack an egg into each one of these indents. Then put the lid back on and cook for 4–6 minutes until the eggs are cooked to your liking.
5. Remove the contents of pan into a bowl and serve with flat parsley if you like.

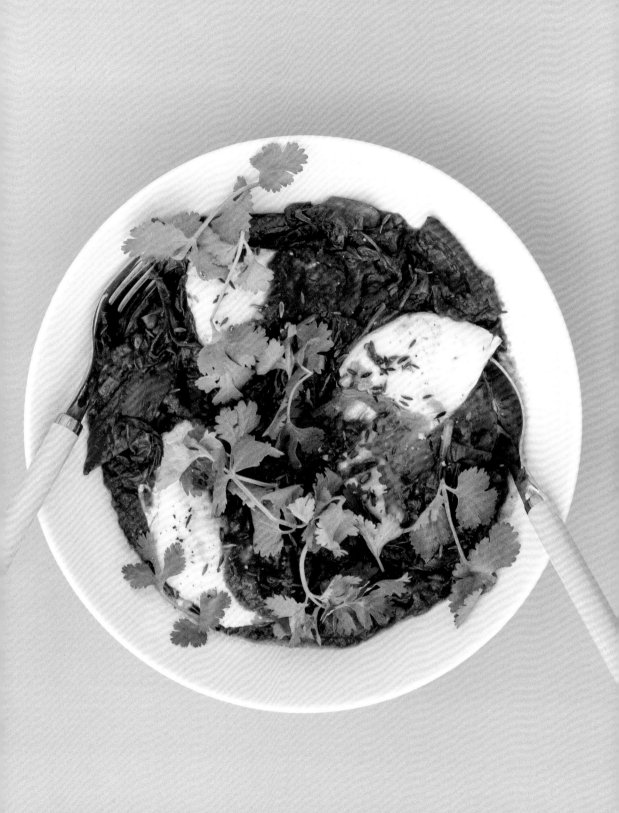

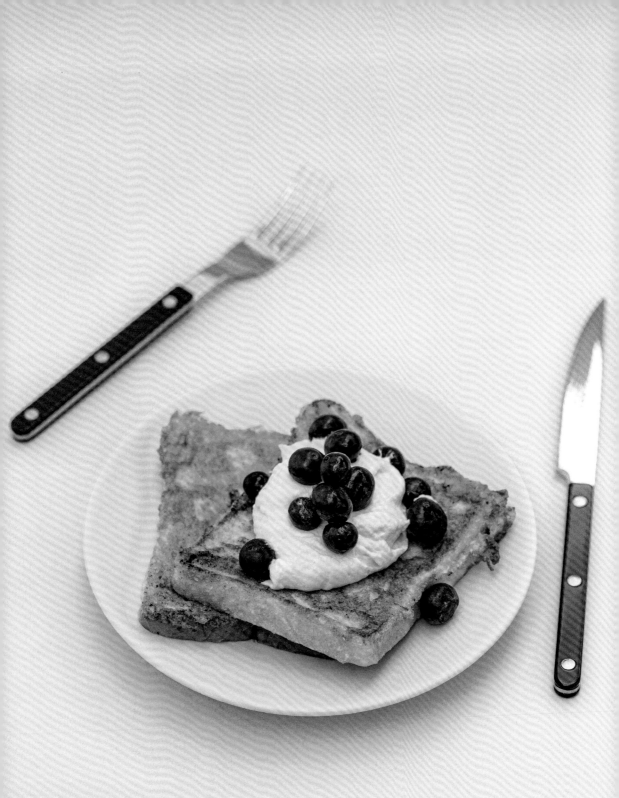

VANILLA & BLUEBERRY
FRENCH TOAST

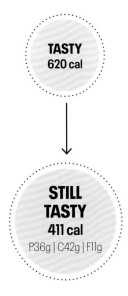

TASTY
620 cal

STILL TASTY
411 cal
P36g | C42g | F11g

French toast is undeniably delicious but often packed with calories. My equally tasty version swaps the 20ml olive oil used to fry the bread with 20 sprays of oil and switches 100g Greek yogurt with 0% fat Greek yogurt for the topping to slash 209 calories without sacrificing any of the flavour!

TAKES 10 minutes

30 × sprays olive oil cooking spray
1 medium egg
2 × 40g slices of white or wholemeal bread

100g 0% fat Greek yogurt
15g vanilla whey protein powder
30g frozen blueberries

1. Spray a large saucepan with the oil and set over a high heat.
2. Crack the egg into a large bowl and beat with a fork until smooth.
3. Dip both sides of the bread in the beaten egg until completely soaked.
4. Place the soaked bread in the pan and fry for 2 minutes on each side.
5. While the bread is cooking, mix the yogurt and protein powder together in a small bowl until evenly combined.
6. Remove the cooked French toast from the pan and top with the yogurt.
7. Tip the blueberries into a heatproof bowl and microwave on full power for 20–30 seconds. Spoon on top of the yogurt and serve.

BERRY & GRANOLA
PROTEIN YOGURT BOWL

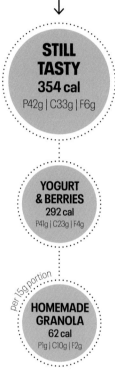

TASTY
512 cal

STILL TASTY
354 cal
P42g | C33g | F6g

YOGURT & BERRIES
292 cal
P41g | C23g | F4g

per 15g portion

HOMEMADE GRANOLA
62 cal
P1g | C10g | F2g

Granola bowls are often highly nutritious, but most granola brands are high in calories, meaning that portion sizes have to be quite small. By making your own version with a few simple ingredients and swapping 250g Greek yogurt for the same amount of 0% fat Greek yogurt you can save 158 calories while still enjoying a nutrient-dense breakfast bowl with a sweet crunch.

TAKES 30 minutes

250g 0% fat Greek yogurt
30g vanilla whey protein powder
30g raspberries
30g blueberries
30g cherries

**For the granola
(Makes 8 servings)**
60g rolled oats
5ml olive oil
10g walnuts, crushed
10g runny honey
30ml maple syrup

1. Preheat the oven to 170°C.
2. Put all the granola ingredients in a large bowl and mix thoroughly with your hands.
3. Line a large, shallow baking tray with baking parchment and spread the granola evenly across the tray. Bake for 12–16 minutes until golden and crunchy. Leave to cool for 5–10 minutes before breaking up. Store in an airtight container in a cool, dark cupboard for up to 3 months.
4. Mix the yogurt and protein powder together in a medium bowl until smooth.
5. Add the berries to the yogurt. Sprinkle over 15g homemade granola and serve.

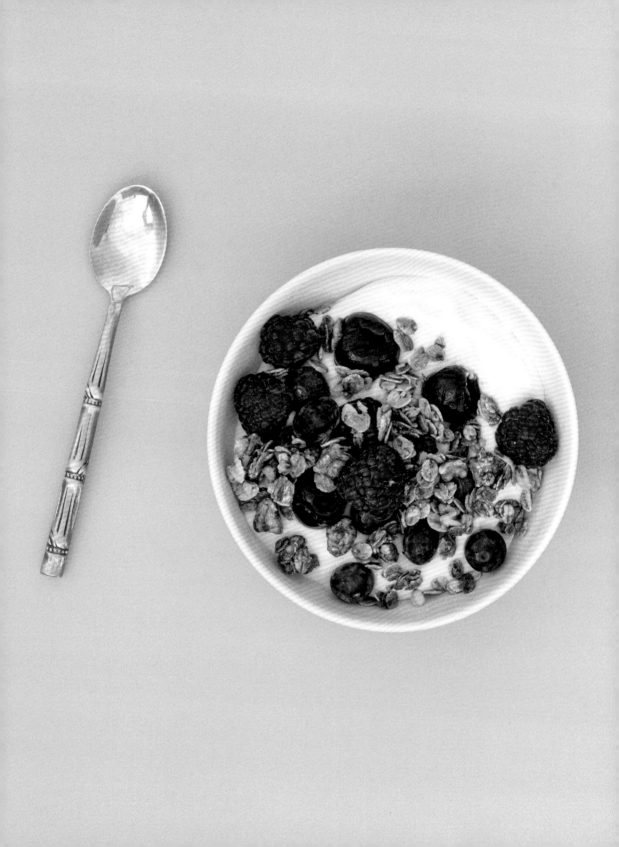

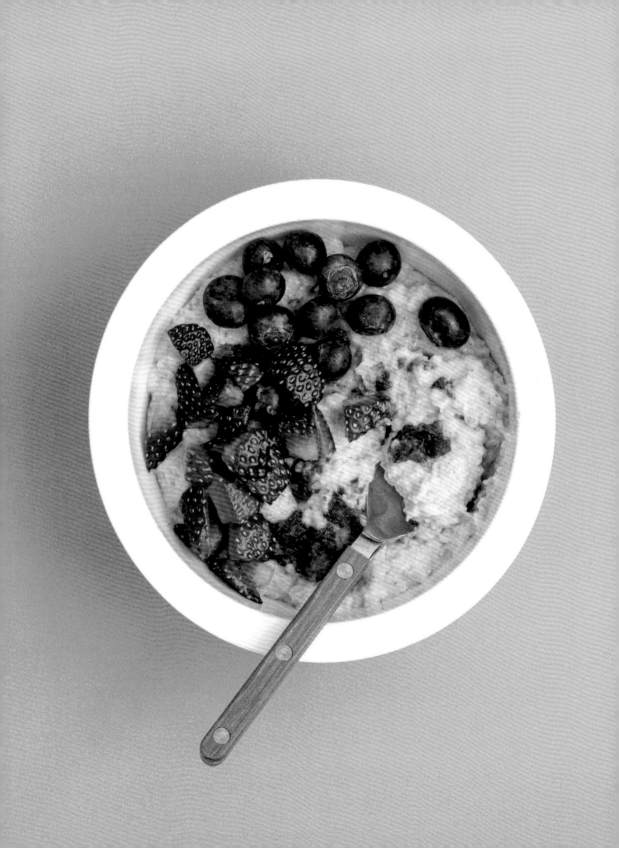

SALTED CARAMEL
PORRIDGE

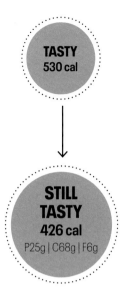

TASTY
530 cal

STILL TASTY
426 cal
P25g | C68g | F6g

Porridge is an age-old, fibre-rich breakfast that is the perfect filling base for many tasty toppings. Despite being nutritious, we often add too much topping, unknowingly increasing the calories in our breakfast. Ditch the 30g caramel syrup for 30g dates, water and salt to enjoy a delicious, low-calorie topping and switch 200ml whole milk for skimmed to reduce the calories without losing any of the flavour. Easy swaps and a saving of 104 calories.

READY IN 5 minutes

50g rolled oats
200ml skimmed milk
20g vanilla whey protein powder
25g pitted dates

20ml water
Pinch of salt
30g blueberries
30g strawberries, hulled and sliced

1. Add the oats and milk to a heatproof bowl and microwave on full power for 2–3 minutes or until the mixture starts to bubble.
2. Remove from the microwave and stir in the protein powder with a tablespoon until smooth.
3. While the oats are cooling, add the dates, water and salt to a blender and blitz until you have a chunky purée. Scrape the purée out of the blender with a wooden spoon and mix into the oats.
4. Top the porridge with the berries and serve.

MAIN MEALS

Many in the fitness industry claim that eating smaller meals more regularly throughout the day assists weight loss. But despite some studies supporting this idea, there is simply no substantiated evidence across a wide range of studies to back this up.

For example, if there were two identical individuals, one consuming 1,800 calories a day across six small meals, the other also consuming 1,800 calories but from two larger meals, there is no evidence to show that there would be any fat-loss benefit to either person. As with breakfast (see page 18), do what suits you. If you prefer eating more smaller meals, do that. If you like eating fewer, larger meals, do so. The important thing to focus on is the total calories you are eating over a period of time.

The lunches and dinners in this section cover a variety of cuisines. Many of the original versions of these dishes are very calorie dense. But that doesn't mean you can't eat them. In fact, I encourage you to enjoy the tasty versions of many of your favourite meals. However, if fat loss is your goal, as you need to reduce the amount of calories you consume, my versions offer you a very similar-tasting, lower calorie alternative that you can eat more regularly.

CROQUE MADAME

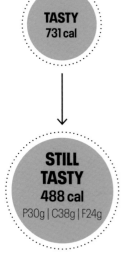

TASTY
731 cal

↓

STILL TASTY
488 cal
P30g | C38g | F24g

Bread, cheese and ham cooked in butter are usually red flags if you're trying to lose weight, but this recipe proves that doesn't have to be the case. All you need to do is reduce the butter from 15g to 10g, the sourdough slices from 60g to 40g and halve the Emmental cheese and you can still enjoy this classic toasted sandwich while saving 243 calories!

TAKES 10 minutes

2 x 40g slices of sourdough
25g Emmental cheese, grated
25g Parma ham slices
10g salted butter

1 medium egg
Black pepper
2 chives stems, chopped

1. Take one of the sourdough slices and place the grated cheese and Parma ham on top. Put the other slice of sourdough on top, pressing the sandwich closed with a spatula.
2. Butter the outsides of the sourdough sandwich.
3. Put a small frying pan over a medium heat. Add the sandwich and fry for 1–2 minutes on each side.
4. Remove the sandwich from the pan and keep warm in an oven heated to 80°C.
5. Crack the egg into the same pan, using the butter residue to fry the egg for 3–5 minutes or until cooked to your liking.
6. Top your toasted sandwich with the fried egg and chives and serve with a twist of black pepper.

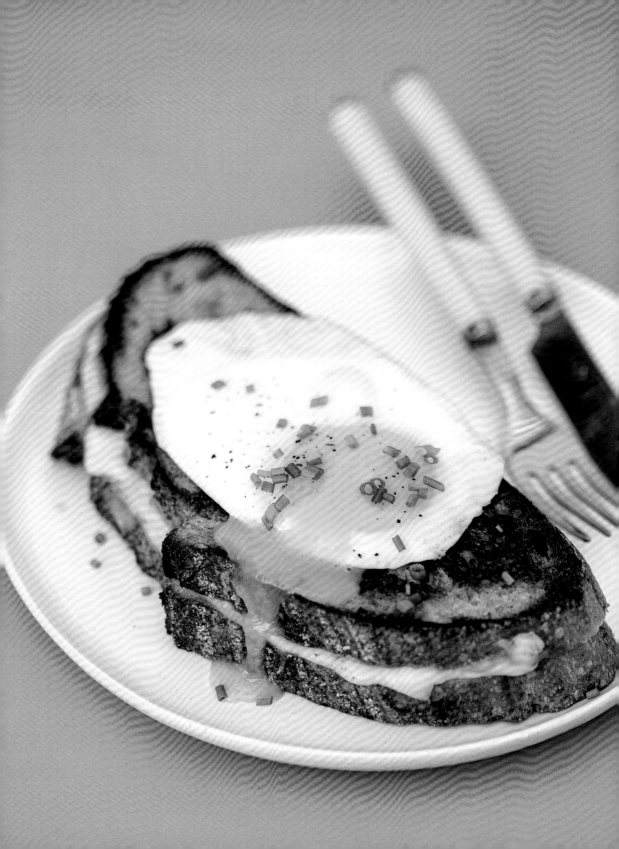

REUBEN
SANDWICH

TASTY
747 cal

STILL
TASTY
509 cal
P33g | C47g | F21g

This much-loved lunch is usually packed full of calories. But with my simple swaps you can still support your calorie deficit and enjoy a delicious Reuben sandwich. Just reduce your regular 60g sourdough slices to 40g, 10g butter to 5g, spread thinly, and use 50% reduced-fat Cheddar cheese alongside light mayonnaise. Exactly the same tasty flavours, but for 238 fewer calories.

TAKES 10 minutes

2 × 40g slices of sourdough
10g unsalted butter, softened
50g pastrami slices
30g 50% reduced-fat Cheddar cheese, grated
30g sauerkraut

For the Russian dressing
15g light mayonnaise
5g tomato ketchup
5ml Worcestershire sauce
Sprinkle of paprika
Salt and pepper

1. Put all the Russian dressing ingredients in a medium bowl and mix well with a fork until evenly combined.
2. Butter both slices of sourdough. Take one slice and add the pastrami, grated cheese and sauerkraut to the non-buttered side.
3. Top with the Russian dressing, then add the remaining sourdough slice, buttered-side up.
4. Heat a medium frying pan over a medium-high heat for 30 seconds, then carefully add the sandwich. Fry for 2–3 minutes on each side until the cheese has melted and the sourdough has become golden and crispy. Serve.

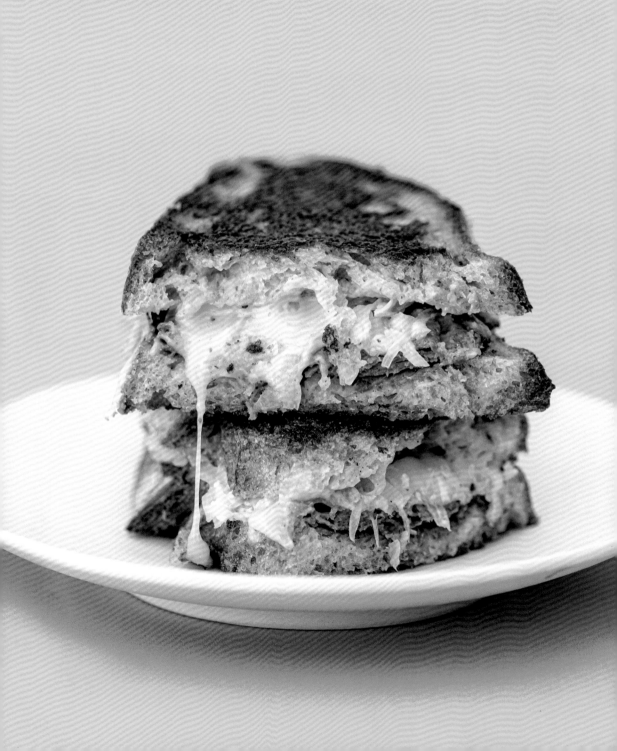

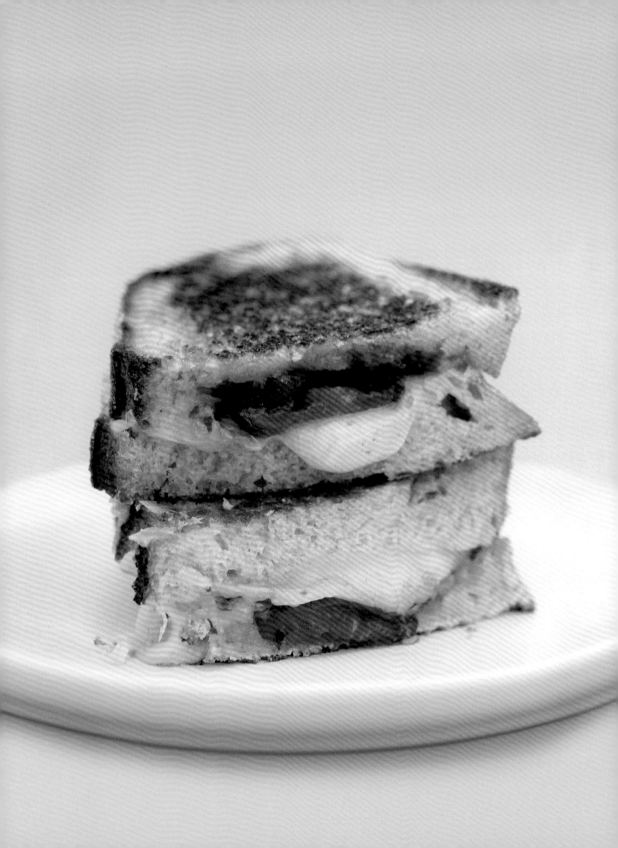

CHEESE, TOMATO
& CHILLI JAM TOASTIE

You can further reduce the calories in this cheese toastie by just replacing the regular Cheddar with a reduced-fat version. The same helping of great-tasting cheese, but with a difference of 103 calories, helping you towards your weight-loss goal. Look out for the chilli jam, too, it's a winning combo!

TAKES 15 minutes

2 × 40g slices of sourdough
60g reduced-fat Cheddar cheese, grated
1 tomato, sliced
5g unsalted butter

For the chilli jam
1 red chilli, deseeded and roughly chopped
10ml passata
10g light soft brown sugar
10ml balsamic vinegar

1. To make the chilli jam, put the red chilli, passata, sugar and balsamic vinegar in a blender or food processor and blitz until smooth. Pour into a small saucepan and heat gently over a low heat for 5–7 minutes, stirring regularly with a wooden spoon, until the mixture bubbles and reduces to a caramelized jam texture.
2. Top one slice of bread with the cheese and tomato before spooning over the chilli jam. Add the remaining slice of bread and press down with spatula.
3. Butter both outsides of the toastie and then place in a small frying pan over a medium heat. Fry for 2–3 minutes on each side until the cheese has melted and the bread has become golden and crispy. Serve.

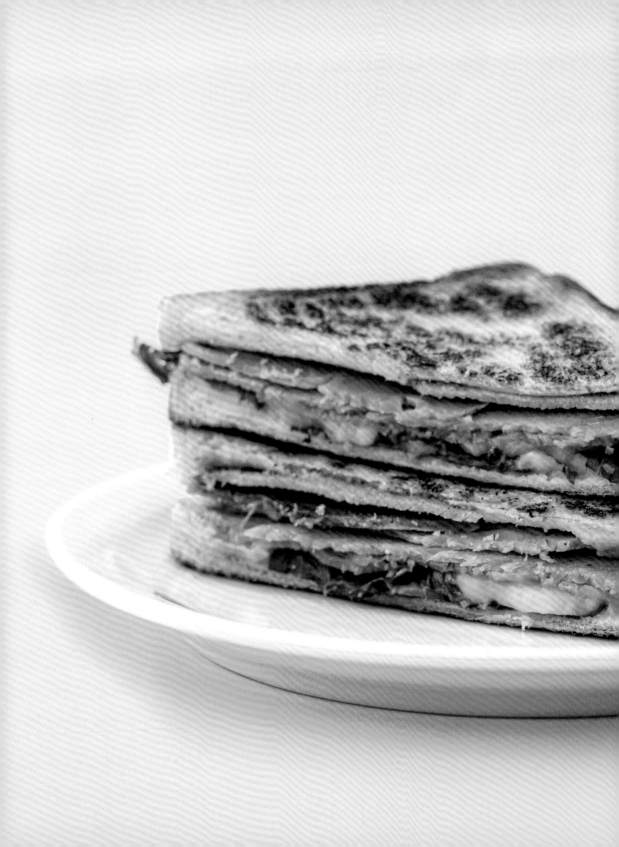

HAM, CHEESE
& SPINACH TOASTIE

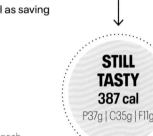

TASTY
500 cal

STILL
TASTY
387 cal
P37g | C35g | F11g

This super-speedy toastie recipe reduces the calories even further by leaving out the butter and dry frying instead of using oil. You also get more protein from the cooked ham as well as saving 113 calories.

TAKES 10 minutes

2 × 40g slices of white
or wholemeal bread
40g reduced-fat Cheddar
cheese, grated

75g cooked, sliced ham
Small handful of baby spinach

1. Heat a medium frying pan over a medium heat.
2. Top one slice of bread with the grated cheese, ham and spinach. Add the remaining slice of bread and press down with a spatula.
3. Using the spatula under the sandwich and your hand on top to stabilize, place the sandwich into the pan, then cook for 4 minutes on each side until the cheese has melted and the bread is golden and crispy. Serve.

STEAK SANDWICH

There are many cuts of beef steak, each containing different amounts of calories, so which one you choose has a big impact on the calories in your sandwich. By opting for 200g fillet steak instead of sirloin, 30 sprays of olive oil rather than 20ml and light mayonnaise rather than the regular kind, you can enjoy this tender, succulent steak sandwich, packed with additional toppings, for 288 calories less than the original.

TAKES 15 minutes

200g fillet steak
Paprika, to taste
30 × sprays olive oil cooking spray
¼ onion, finely sliced
90g ciabatta roll

10g Dijon mustard
10g light mayonnaise
Small handful of fresh rocket
Salt and pepper

1. On a chopping board, season both sides of the fillet steak with paprika, salt and pepper.
2. Add 15 sprays of oil to a small saucepan, put over a medium heat, then add the onion and cook for 3 minutes. Add a splash of water to the pan and remove from the heat.
3. Spray a separate small frying pan with 15 sprays of oil, then put over a high heat and sear the steak for 3–5 minutes on each side or until cooked to your liking.
4. While the steak is cooking, cut the ciabatta in half and lightly toast it in a toaster.
5. In a small bowl, mix the mustard and mayonnaise together with a spoon until even, then spread on the ciabatta and fill with the cooked onions and rocket.
6. Finally, remove the cooked steak from the pan and set aside to rest for 2 minutes. Slice and add to the ciabatta. Serve.

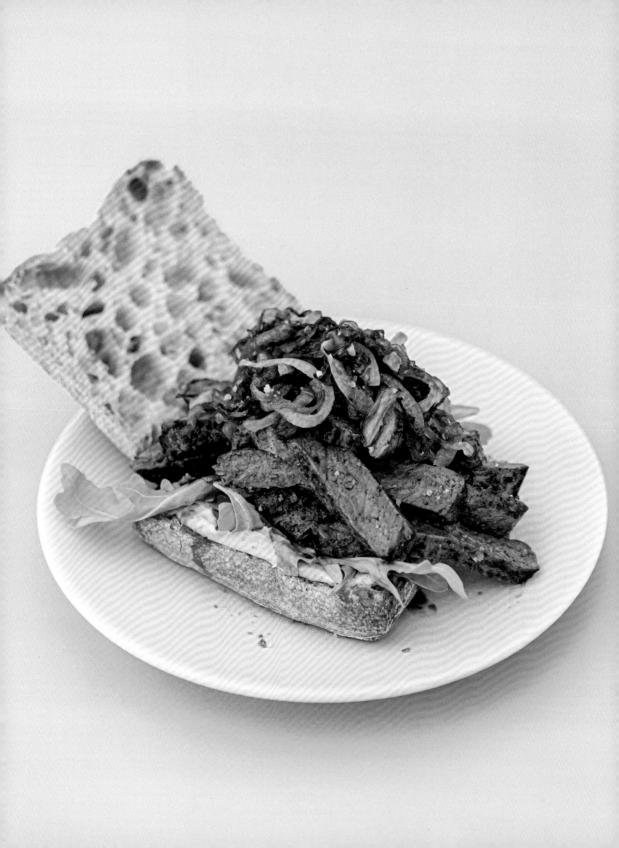

BLT SANDWICH

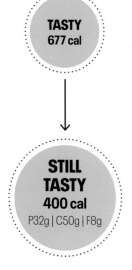

TASTY
677 cal

STILL TASTY
400 cal
P32g | C50g | F8g

This classic sandwich enjoyed by millions is sadly often packed with calories as well as flavour. But by switching bacon rashers for bacon medallions, removing the 5ml cooking oil and grilling the bacon, then using light mayonnaise and cutting thinner slices of sourdough, you can still enjoy all the taste of a BLT while saving 277 calories.

TAKES 10 minutes

4 bacon medallions
2 × 30g slices of sourdough
10g light mayonnaise

1 medium iceberg lettuce leaf
1 tomato, sliced

1. Preheat the grill to high. Put the bacon medallions on a foil-lined baking tray and grill for 4–5 minutes on each side until they begin to look golden and crispy.
2. While the bacon is cooking, evenly spread one slice of sourdough with the mayonnaise, then top with the lettuce and sliced tomato.
3. Add the grilled bacon, top with the remaining slice of sourdough and press down. Cut in half and serve.

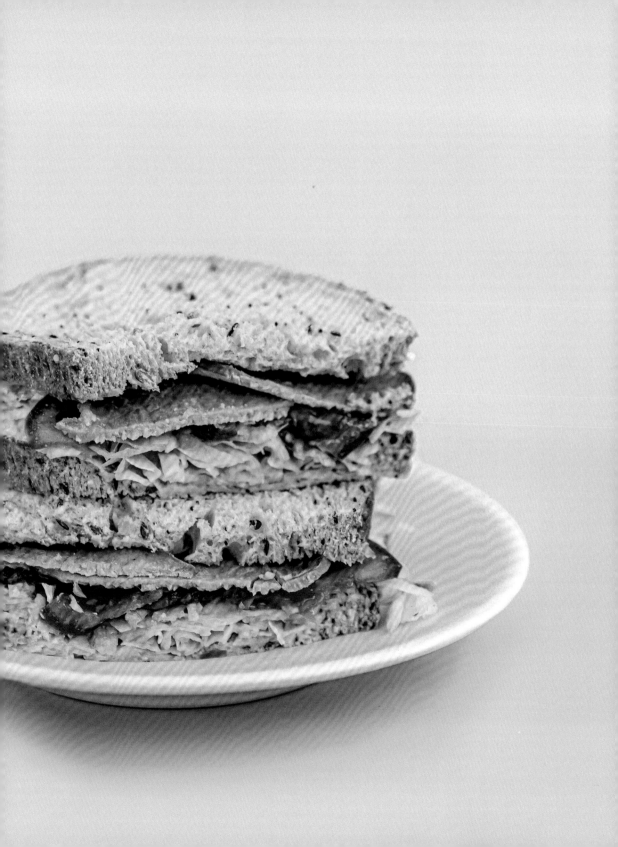

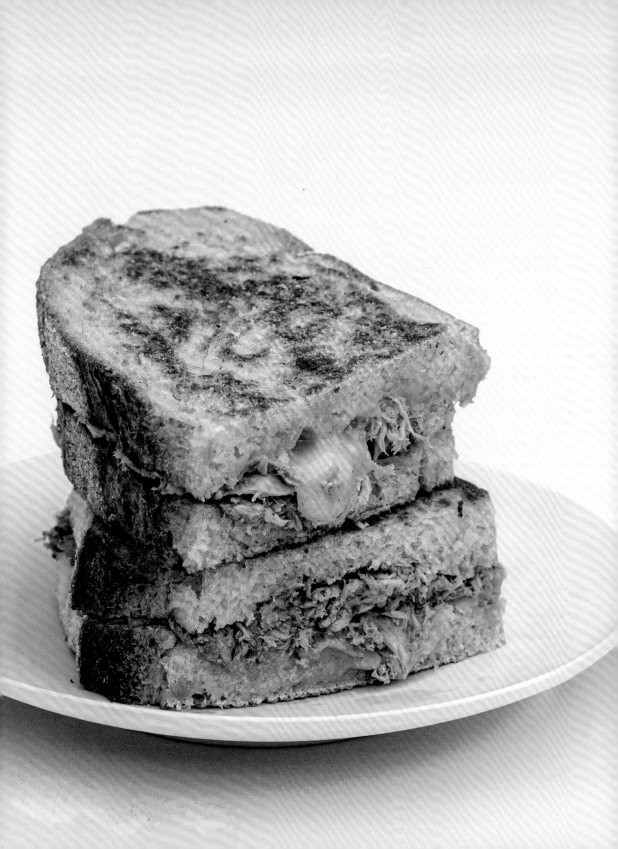

TUNA & RED
PESTO MELT

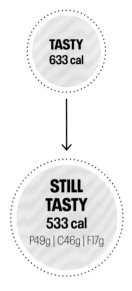

TASTY
633 cal

STILL TASTY
533 cal
P49g | C46g | F17g

The tuna melt is a top lunch choice for many but this one has 100 calories less than most versions. All you need to do is swap the regular pesto and Cheddar for reduced-fat variations. Easy!

TAKES 10 minutes

120g can of tuna (drained weight)
30g 30% reduced-fat Cheddar cheese, grated

30g reduced-fat red pesto
2 × 40g slices of sourdough
10 × sprays of olive oil spray

1. In a small bowl, combine the tuna, cheese and pesto with a fork until evenly mixed.
2. Add the mix evenly to one slice of sourdough before adding the remaining slice on top. Press down with a spatula to seal the edges.
3. Spray a small saucepan with the oil and set over a medium heat.
4. Fry the toastie for 3–5 minutes on each side. Reduce the heat to low if you don't want it too crispy! Serve.

TURKEY MEATBALL SUB

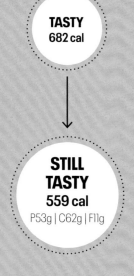

TASTY
682 cal

STILL TASTY
559 cal

P53g | C62g | F11g

The meatball sub is popular around the world, whether it's a takeaway or homemade. If weight loss is your aim, swapping 150g turkey thigh mince for turkey breast mince and 10ml olive oil for 10 sprays of olive oil cooking spray cuts 123 calories, supporting your calorie deficit while losing none of the delicious meatball taste.

TAKES 20 minutes

150g turkey breast mince	¼ onion, finely chopped
10g panko breadcrumbs	10 × sprays olive oil cooking spray
1 medium egg	20g barbecue sauce
10g oats	1 tsp paprika
½ tsp garlic powder	50ml water
½ tsp mild chilli powder	100g sub roll
½ tsp salt	Small handful of baby spinach

1. Put the turkey mince, breadcrumbs, egg, oats, garlic powder, chilli powder, salt and onion in a large bowl. Mix with your hands until thoroughly combined and then form the mixture into 3 evenly sized meatballs.
2. Spray a medium saucepan with the oil spray and set over a medium heat. Sear the meatballs for 5 minutes, moving them around the pan with a spatula until a crust forms.
3. Reduce the heat slightly and cook the meatballs for a further 10 minutes, moving them around the pan regularly.
4. Add the barbecue sauce, paprika and water and mix into the meatballs. Cook for 2–3 minutes or until the sauce begins to bubble.
5. Cut open the sub roll, add the meatballs, sauce and spinach. Serve.

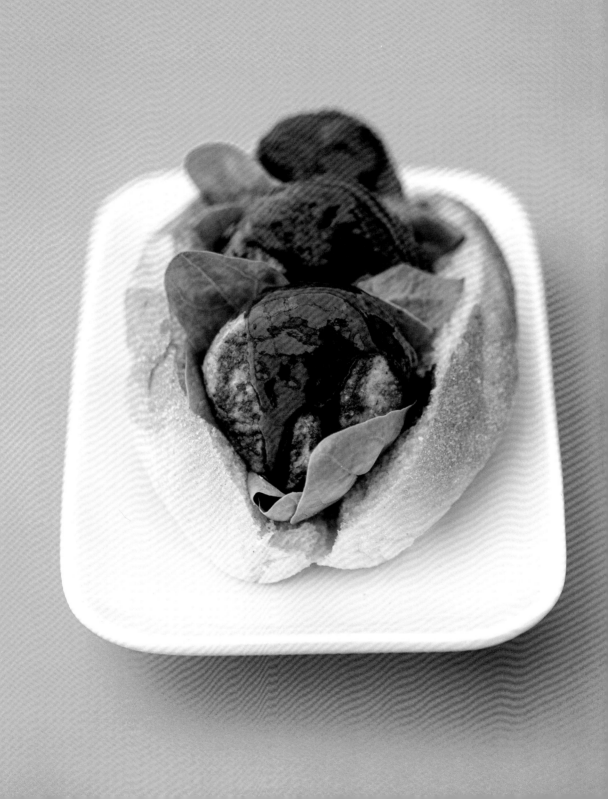

CLUB SANDWICH

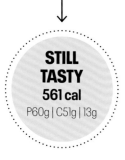

TASTY
741 cal

STILL TASTY
561 cal
P60g | C51g | 13g

To enjoy the same great taste of this sandwich favourite and reduce the calories to help you lose weight, simply switch 4 rashers of streaky bacon for the same amount of turkey bacon and swap in light mayonnaise for the regular version. You save 180 calories with consummate ease.

TAKES 15 minutes

4 rashers of turkey bacon
3 × 40g slices of white or wholemeal bread
15g light mayonnaise
1 tomato, sliced
50g cooked, skinless chicken breast, roughly chopped

Small handful of iceberg lettuce, shredded
1 small slice of Edam cheese
1 large cocktail stick

1. Preheat the grill to high. Put the turkey bacon on a foil-lined tray and grill for 10–12 minutes, turning halfway through cooking.
2. When the turkey bacon is nearly cooked, lightly toast the bread.
3. Spread one slice of bread with half the mayonnaise and top with the grilled turkey bacon, sliced tomato and another slice of bread.
4. Spread the remaining mayonnaise on the second slice of bread, then add the chopped chicken, lettuce and cheese before placing the final slice of bread on top.
5. Spear a large cocktail stick through the centre of the sandwich to keep it intact while cutting into halves or quarters as you please. Serve.

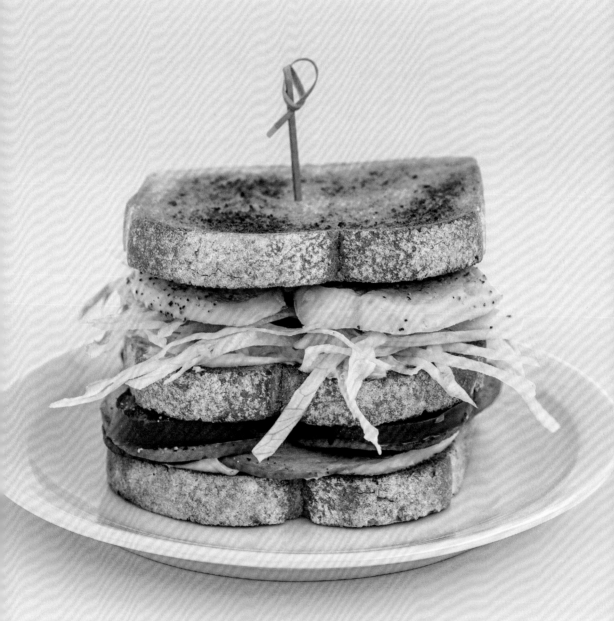

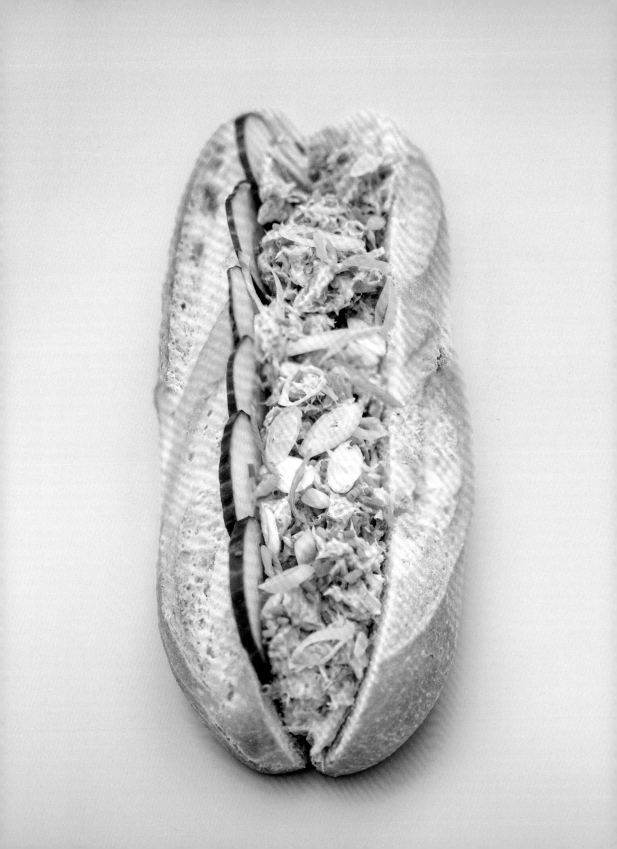

TUNA MAYONNAISE
& CUCUMBER BAGUETTE

TASTY
606 cal

STILL TASTY
474 cal
P38g | 58g | F10g

Tuna mayo is one of the most popular shop-bought sandwich fillings. Here we keep the same amount, but still reduce the calories by using a slightly smaller 100g baguette. Then simply swap the mayonnaise for a light version. If you usually enjoy this lunch three times a week, you'll save 396 calories with this easy adjustment.

TAKES 5 minutes

120g can of tuna (120g drained weight)
30g light mayonnaise
1 spring onion, finely chopped
Small handful of freshly chopped chives

100g baguette
40g cucumber, sliced
Salt and pepper

1. Put the tuna and light mayonnaise in a medium bowl and mix thoroughly with a fork until they form a thick paste.
2. Add the spring onion and chives, season with salt and pepper, and stir together with a fork.
3. Slice open the baguette, then add the tuna mayonnaise and sliced cucumber. Enjoy straightaway or take with you to eat for lunch.

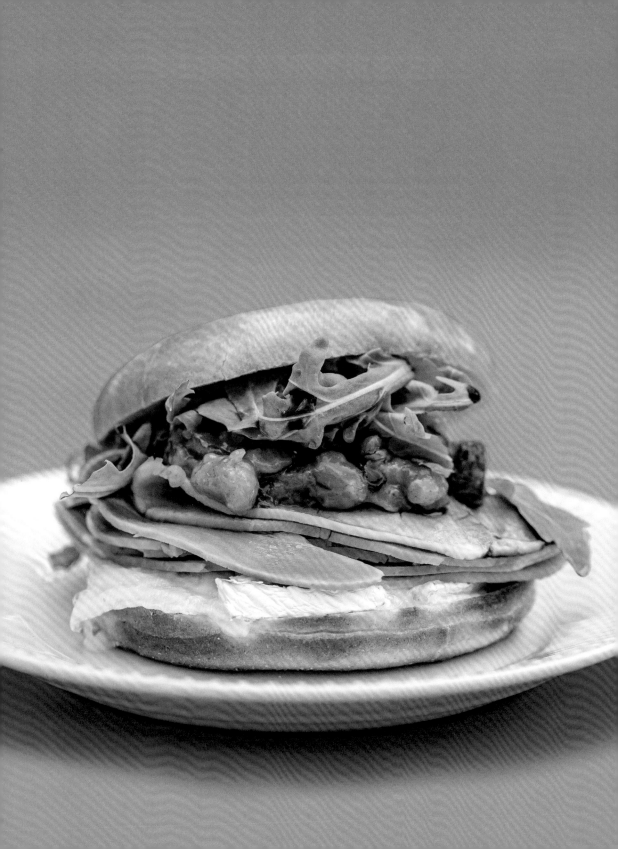

TOASTED BRIE, HAM
& PICKLE BAGEL

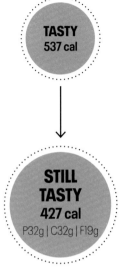

TASTY
537 cal

STILL TASTY
427 cal
P32g | C32g | F19g

Cheese is often demonized as a calorie-dense food which you have to cut out completely if you're trying to lose weight. But by making other easy ingredient swaps to reduce calories, you can still enjoy your favourite cheese without resorting to tiny portions. This recipe uses a bagel thin rather than a standard bagel to save 110 calories. See how simple caloric reduction can be...

TAKES 10 minutes

1 bagel thin
50g brie cheese, sliced
15g your favourite pickle or vegetable chutney

75g cooked ham, cut into thick slices
Small handful of fresh rocket
5ml balsamic vinegar

1. Preheat the grill to medium.
2. Slice the bagel thin in half and add the sliced brie to both halves.
3. Transfer to a foil-lined baking tray and grill for 3–4 minutes until the brie softens and the bagel thin begins to brown.
4. Remove from the grill, then spread the pickle evenly over both halves.
5. Top one bagel half with the sliced ham and rocket before drizzling over the balsamic vinegar. Then place the other bagel half on top. Serve.

ZINGY CHICKEN,
AVOCADO & NACHO WRAP

Wraps are a popular lunchtime choice. but sadly many supermarket versions are small so that they can claim fewer calories on the label. They also tend to load up on dressings and reduce protein like meat and poultry to make production cheaper. Here you won't skimp on the star ingredients – which is why you wanted the wrap in the first place! You can enjoy more chicken and succulent, mashed avocado as well as crunchy nachos by losing the 20g mayonnaise usually smeared in readymade wraps and replacing it with 0% fat Greek yogurt.

TAKES 5 minutes

½ small avocado
Juice of ¼ lime
Twist of salt
Sprinkle of garlic powder
1 medium tortilla wrap
10g 0% fat Greek yogurt
75g cooked, skinless chicken breast, cut into 3cm pieces

Small handful of chopped round lettuce
¼ yellow pepper, finely chopped
1 tbsp finely chopped red onion
3 tortilla chips (spicy flavour works best), crushed
Dash of sriracha sauce

1. Mash the avocado in a small bowl. Add the lime juice, salt and garlic powder, mix and spread over the tortilla wrap.
2. Spread the Greek yogurt evenly on the tortilla wrap. Then fill it with the chicken, red onion, lettuce, yellow pepper and crushed tortilla chips. Drizzle the sriracha sauce over the top.
3. Tuck in the edges of the wrap. Then quickly flip over the wrap to ensure filling is secure. Slice down the middle and serve.

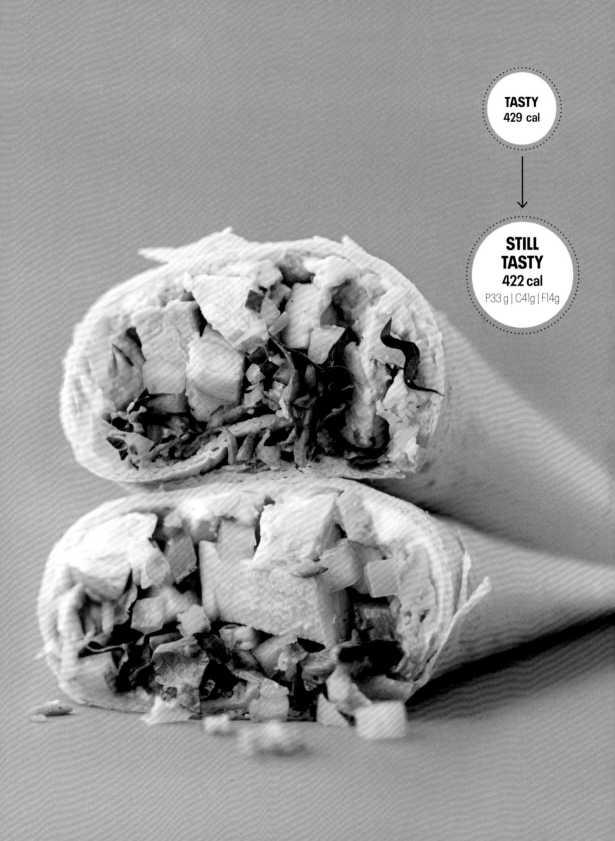

TASTY
429 cal

STILL
TASTY
422 cal
P33 g | C41g | F14g

TEX-MEX CHICKEN WRAP

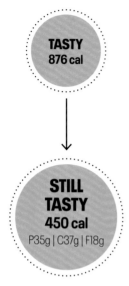

TASTY
876 cal

STILL
TASTY
450 cal
P35g | C37g | F18g

By taking the skin off the chicken thighs, swapping 10ml cooking oil for 10 sprays of olive oil cooking spray and 10ml flavoured mayonnaise for 10ml hot sauce mixed with 30g 0% fat Greek yogurt, you can enjoy the same Tex-Mex tastes and textures of your favourite chicken wrap, but also save a massive 426 calories.

TAKES 20 minutes

10 × sprays olive oil cooking spray
¼ red pepper, sliced
¼ red onion, sliced
1 medium tortilla wrap
1 large leaf round lettuce, chopped
10ml hot sauce
30g 0% fat Greek yogurt
Salt and pepper

For the Tex-Mex chicken
150g skinless, boneless chicken thighs
½ tsp paprika
½ tsp ground cumin
½ tsp garlic powder
½ tsp mild chilli powder
½ tsp salt
5g plain flour
Juice of ½ lemon
Sprinkle of chipotle chilli flakes

1. Preheat the grill to high.
2. Put all the ingredients for the Tex-Mex chicken in a large bowl and mix together with your hands until evenly combined.
3. Transfer the chicken to a small, foil-lined baking dish and grill for 6–7 minutes on each side.
4. While the chicken thighs are cooking, spray a small frying pan with the oil and set over a medium heat. Add the pepper and onion with a little seasoning and fry for 6–7 minutes until softened.
5. Chop the grilled chicken into small strips, then add to the centre of the tortilla wrap with the lettuce and cooked pepper and onion.
6. Mix the hot sauce together with the Greek yogurt in a small bowl until evenly coloured, then spoon over the top of the other ingredients. Roll into a wrap, chop down the centre and serve.

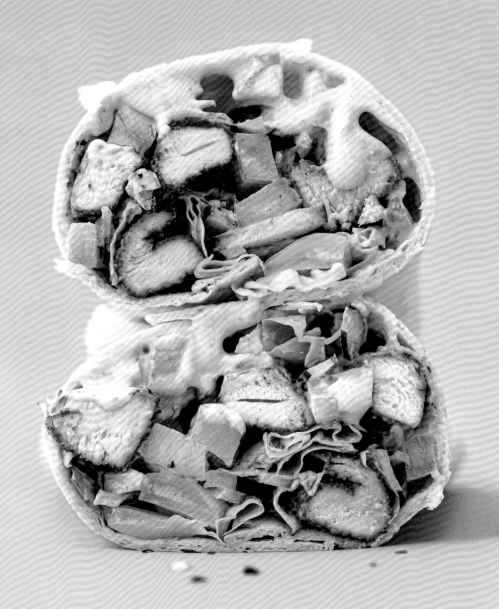

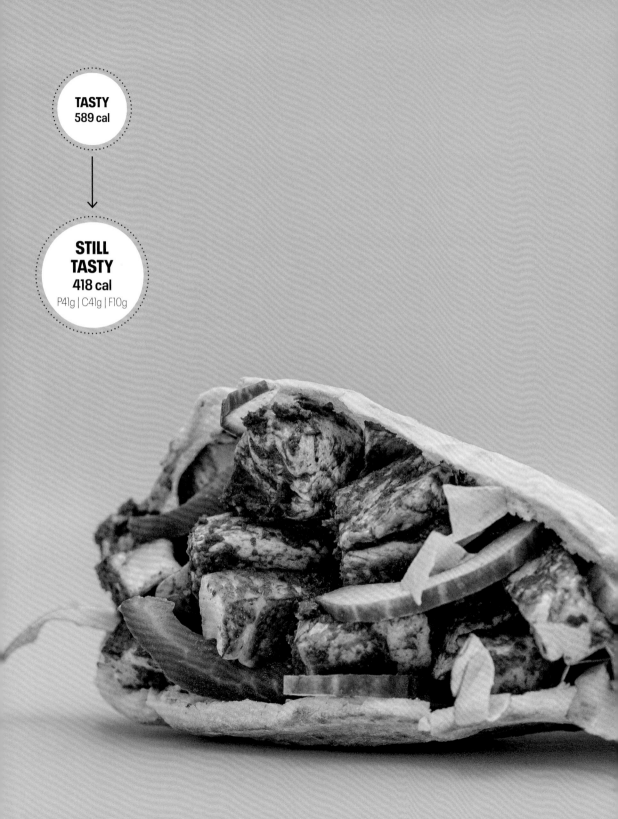

TASTY
589 cal

**STILL
TASTY**
418 cal
P41g | C41g | F10g

PERI-PERI CHICKEN
& HALLOUMI PITTA

Many marinades contain large quantities of oil, increasing the overall calories in the dish. Here you leave out the 20ml oil usually used to marinate and cook the chicken and use 10 sprays of olive oil cooking spray instead. The same Peri-peri flavours but with 171 fewer calories.

TAKES 20 minutes

10 × sprays olive oil cooking spray
125g skinless chicken breast, chopped into 3cm pieces
20g halloumi, sliced
1 medium pitta
Small handful of sliced round lettuce
2 slices of tomato
30g cucumber, sliced

For the Peri-peri marinade
2 small red chillies, deseeded and roughly chopped
50ml cider vinegar
3 garlic cloves
1 tbsp smoked paprika
Juice from ½ lemon
Small handful of flat-leaf parsley
Pinch of salt

1. Put all the marinade ingredients in a blender or food processor and blitz until smooth.
2. Spray a medium saucepan with the oil and set over a medium heat. Add the chicken and cook for 5 minutes.
3. Reduce the heat slightly, add the marinade and stir in with the chicken. Cook for a further 10 minutes until the sauce has reduced to a paste. If it's looking too dry, add a dash of water and stir.
4. While the chicken is cooking, put a separate small frying or griddle pan over a medium heat, add the halloumi slices and sear for 2 minutes on each side until dark brown.
5. Slice open the pitta and add the chicken, halloumi, lettuce, tomato and cucumber. Serve.

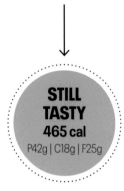

TASTY
730 cal

STILL TASTY
465 cal
P42g | C18g | F25g

CHICKEN CAESAR
SALAD

This salad is always a favourite, wherever you are in the world. Most recipes include a calorie-dense dressing rich in mayonnaise, olive oil and Parmesan. But you can still get the same great taste using smaller amounts of ingredients. By reducing the usual 20ml olive oil to 10ml, 50g Parmesan to 25g and swapping the mayonnaise for a light version, you save a significant 265 calories, but still enjoy the same classic Caesar flavours.

TAKES 5 minutes

125g cooked, skinless chicken breast, cut into 3cm pieces
25g croutons (seasoned to your choice)
1 tsp garlic powder
½ tsp salt
½ tsp black pepper
Juice of ¼ lemon
1 small Romaine lettuce, chopped
20g Parmesan shavings

For the Caesar dressing
5g capers, drained
½ tsp garlic purée
15g light mayonnaise
½ tsp Dijon mustard
Juice of ¼ lemon
5g Parmesan cheese, grated
10ml olive oil

1. Put the chicken and croutons in a large bowl along with the garlic powder, salt, black pepper and lemon juice. Mix with your hands until the chicken is evenly seasoned.
2. To make the Caesar dressing, put the capers on a chopping board, place a piece of clingfilm over the top and mash into a paste with the end of a rolling pin. Add the paste to a small bowl with the remaining dressing ingredients and stir with a fork until evenly combined.
3. Transfer the seasoned chicken and croutons to a large serving dish, add the chopped lettuce, Parmesan shavings and Caesar dressing and mix well before serving.

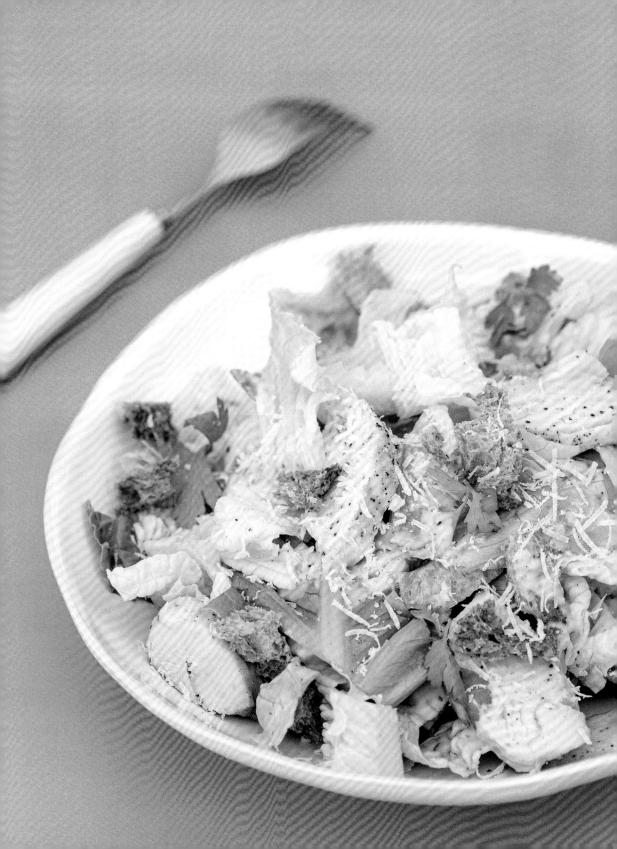

ZESTY SMOKED SALMON
& FETA PASTA SALAD

This recipe is extremely easy to make and ideal for taking to work and storing in the fridge until it's time to tuck in. You don't need shop-bought dressings to add flavour here. Just use lemon juice, plus salt and pepper for a refreshing taste, saving 80 calories in the process.

TAKES 15 minutes

50g uncooked penne
75g smoked salmon, sliced into 2cm strips
5 cherry tomatoes, halved
Small handful of baby spinach
40g cucumber, chopped into small chunks

25g feta cheese, chopped into small chunks
Juice from ½ lemon
Salt and pepper

1. Fill a small saucepan with water and bring to the boil. Add the penne and cook for 6–8 minutes until tender; test with a fork. Rinse the penne in cold water for 30 seconds, then drain.
2. While the penne is cooking, put the smoked salmon, cherry tomatoes, spinach, cucumber and feta in a serving bowl and mix thoroughly with your hands.
3. Add the cooled penne, lemon juice, salt and some black pepper and toss with your hands. Serve or transfer to a Tupperware container to enjoy the next day. Store in the fridge.

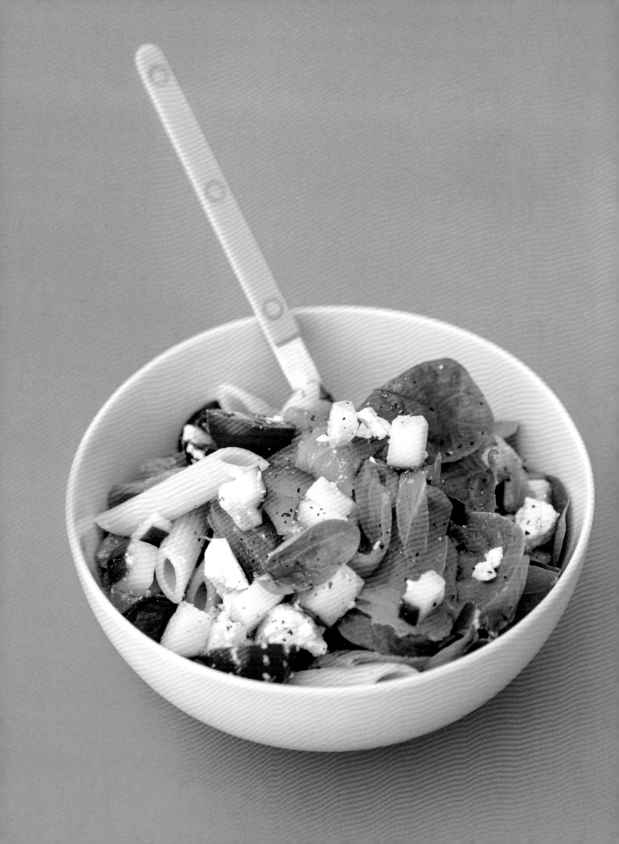

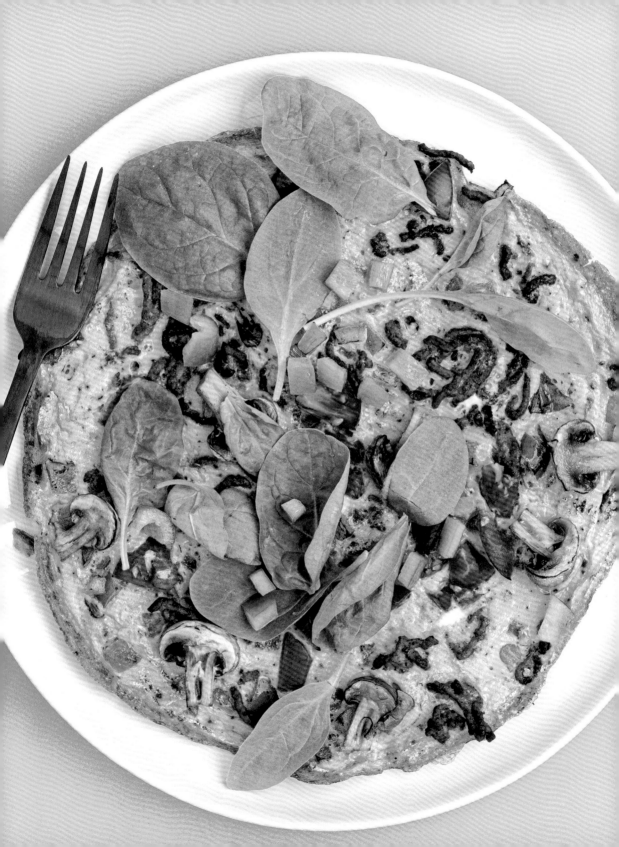

BEEF & MUSHROOM
OMELETTE

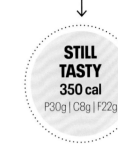

TASTY
485 cal

STILL
TASTY
350 cal
P30g | C8g | F22g

By reducing the usual 20ml cooking oil for this omelette to 5ml, you can save 135 calories and enjoy the same-sized portion and flavours.

READY IN 5 minutes

5ml olive oil
3 medium eggs
3 medium button mushrooms
50g 5% fat beef mince

¼ red onion, finely chopped
½ green pepper, finely chopped
1 tomato, finely chopped
Salt and pepper

1. Put a medium saucepan over a high heat and add the olive oil. Tilt the pan to spread the oil evenly over the base of the pan.
2. Crack the eggs into a small bowl, add the remaining ingredients, season with salt and pepper and whisk with a fork until evenly combined.
3. Add the egg mixture to the pan and allow it to set for 20–30 seconds. Then manoeuvre the pan in a circular motion and lift up the cooked egg with a spatula to allow the uncooked egg underneath to cook. Repeat for 3–4 minutes until all the egg mixture is fully cooked.
4. Season with more salt and pepper and garnish with baby spinach, if you wish. Serve.

LOADED CHORIZO
ROLL-UP OMELETTE

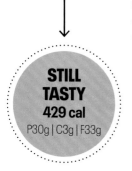

The 135 calories you save by reducing 20ml olive oil to 5ml means you can add even more tasty toppings. This recipe combines delicious goat's cheese and chorizo in a rolled-up omelette variation.

TAKES 10 minutes

5ml olive oil	20g goat's cheese, crumbled
3 medium eggs	20g chorizo, sliced
¼ red pepper, finely chopped	30ml passata
½ tsp salt	½ tsp dried basil
½ tsp black pepper	1 medium tortilla wrap
½ tsp dried oregano	

1. Put a medium saucepan over a high heat and add the olive oil. Tilt the pan to spread the oil evenly over the base of the pan.
2. Crack the eggs into a small bowl, then add the red pepper, salt, pepper and oregano and beat with a fork until smooth.
3. Add the egg mixture to the pan and allow it to set for 20–30 seconds. Then manoeuvre the pan in a circular motion and lift up the cooked egg with a spatula to allow the uncooked egg underneath to cook. Repeat for 3–4 minutes until all the egg mixture is nearly cooked.
4. Scatter over the crumbled goat's cheese and sliced chorizo, reduce the heat to low and cook for 2 minutes.
5. Mix the passata and basil together in a small bowl and spread over the tortilla wrap. Transfer the tortilla to a microwave-safe plate and heat on full power for 30 seconds.
6. Remove the cooked omelette from the pan with a spatula and place on top of the tortilla, then roll up and serve.

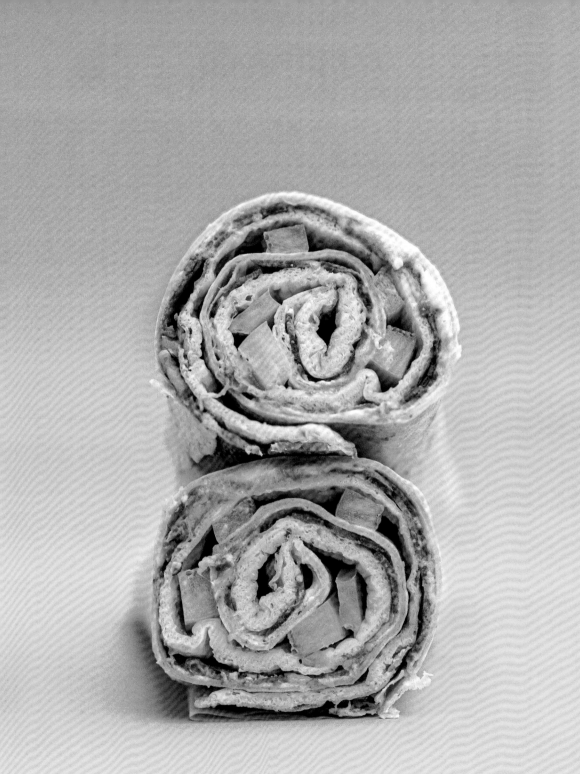

BAKED POTATO
with cheese, tangy beans & chorizo

Baked potatoes are versatile, easy-to-prep meals. You can top them with a variety of fillings to suit your tastes and dietary needs, but a popular choice is always calorie-dense cheese and baked beans. Rather than banning your favourite ingredients, it's better to change them slightly so you can still enjoy the same tasty meals. Here, by just swapping the Cheddar for a 50% reduced-fat version and removing the 15g butter often melted into the potato, you can save 168 calories and savour a simple dinner using only five ingredients. You also save a lot of time microwaving the potato instead of baking it.

TAKES 15 minutes

400g baking potato
150g baked beans
15ml Worcestershire sauce
1 tsp dried Italian herbs
10g diced chorizo

10g 50% reduced-fat crème fraîche
5g barbecue sauce
2 chives, freshly chopped
30g 50% reduced-fat Cheddar
   cheese, grated

1. Prick the potato all over with a fork before placing on a microwave-safe dish. Microwave on full power for 7–10 minutes. Turn over halfway through cooking. When the potato is soft enough to pierce easily with a knife it is ready.
2. While the potato is cooking, put the baked beans, Worcestershire sauce and Italian herbs in a small saucepan. Heat gently over a low heat for 3–5 minutes, stirring with a wooden spoon.
3. Cut a cross in the cooked potato to open it up (careful – it's hot). Then add the tangy beans, chorizo, crème fraîche, chives, barbecue sauce and grated cheese. Microwave for a further 30 seconds–1 minute if you want the cheese to melt quickly. Serve.

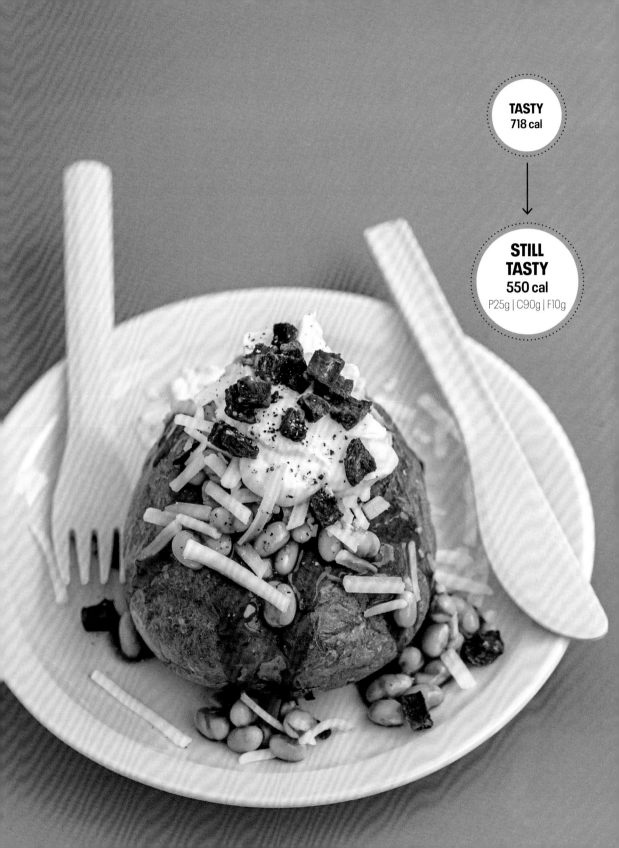

TASTY
718 cal

STILL
TASTY
550 cal
P25g | C90g | F10g

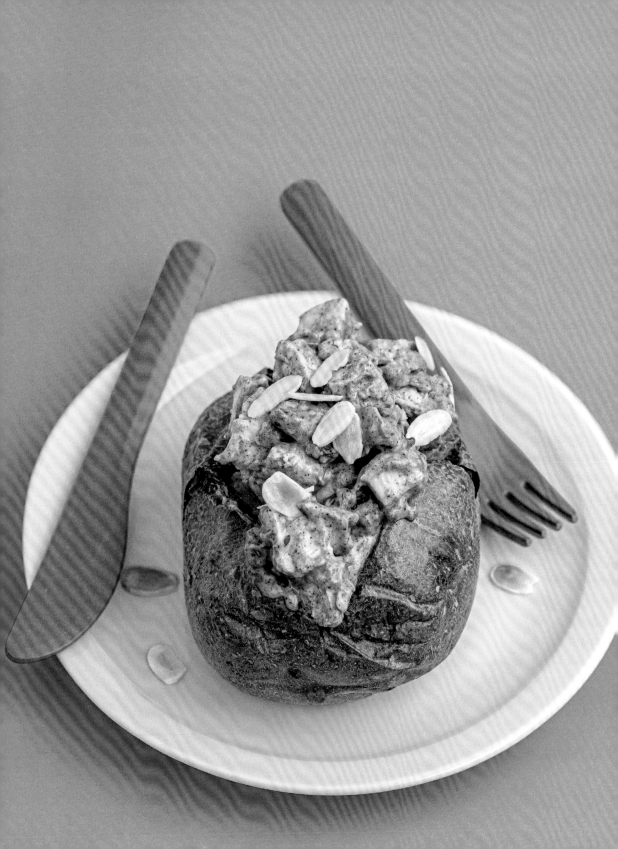

CORONATION CHICKEN
BAKED POTATO

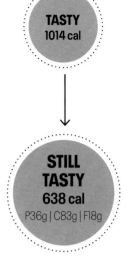

TASTY
1014 cal

STILL TASTY
638 cal
P36g | C83g | F18g

Most of the calories in this baked-potato favourite come from the coronation sauce. But by simply swapping the mayonnaise for half-fat crème fraîche, reducing the olive oil from 10ml to 5ml and ditching the usual 10g butter melted into the potato, you save 376 calories and can still enjoy the same flavours without having to reduce your portion size.

TAKES 55 minutes

400g baking potato
5ml olive oil
100g skinless chicken breast, chopped into 3cm pieces
50g half-fat crème fraîche
½ tsp ground cinnamon

½ tsp curry powder
10g sultanas
15g mango chutney
5g toasted almond flakes
Black pepper

1. Preheat the oven to 200°C.
2. Prick the potato all over with a fork before placing in a small baking dish. Bake for 45 minutes until soft enough to pierce easily with a knife, but crispy on the outside.
3. While the potato is cooking, put a small saucepan over a medium heat. Add the olive oil, a pinch of black pepper and the chicken and cook for 10 minutes until cooked through. Set aside to cool.
4. To make the coronation sauce, put the crème fraîche, cinnamon, curry powder, sultanas, mango chutney and almond flakes in a small bowl and mix with a fork until evenly combined.
5. Add the cooled chicken to the coronation sauce, mix and chill until the potato is baked.
6. Cut a cross in the cooked potato to open it up. Then add the coronation chicken and serve.

PATATAS BRAVAS

TASTY
710 cal

STILL TASTY
458 cal
P11g | C72g | F14g

This recipe transforms the simple, classic tapas dish into a versatile main meal. You roast/grill the potatoes instead of deep-frying them to keep the crispiness but with significantly fewer calories. In addition, swapping the soured cream for a low-fat version saves 252 calories while maintaining the classic textures and tastes of the original.

TAKES 55 minutes

10 × sprays olive oil cooking spray
10ml olive oil
350g potatoes, cut into thumb-sized pieces
200g canned chopped tomatoes
¼ onion, finely chopped
1 tsp garlic powder
1 tsp hot paprika

1 tsp smoked paprika
1 red chilli, roughly chopped and blitzed with 10ml water
20g low-fat soured cream
Small bunch of finely chopped flat-leaf parsley
Salt

1. Preheat the oven to 220°C. Line a large, shallow baking tray with foil and spray evenly with the oil.
2. Pour the 10ml olive oil into a large bowl, then add the potatoes and a pinch of salt and mix thoroughly with your hands to make sure they are completely coated in the oil. Transfer the potatoes to the foil-lined tray and roast for 40–45 minutes until golden and crispy. To crisp further, preheat the grill to high and grill for a final 3–4 minutes.
3. While the potatoes are cooking, put a medium saucepan over a medium heat and add the chopped tomatoes, onion, garlic powder, hot paprika, smoked paprika, blitzed red chilli and a pinch of salt. Simmer for 8–10 minutes.
4. Transfer the cooked potatoes to a serving dish, then pour over the tomato bravas sauce and garnish with more salt, soured cream and the chopped parsley.

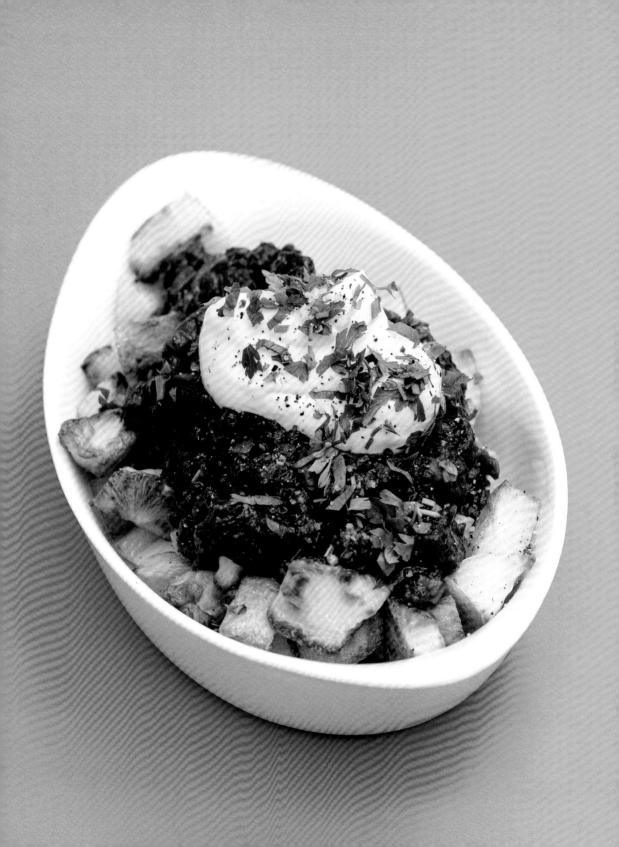

MARGHERITA PIZZA

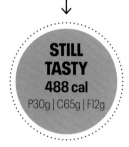

TASTY
581 cal

STILL TASTY
488 cal
P30g | C65g | F12g

You can still enjoy this classic cheese and tomato pizza if you want to lose weight, just swap the mozzarella for a reduced-fat version. A saving of 93 calories and you don't even have to reduce the portion size.

TAKES 25 minutes

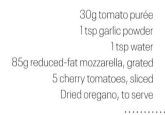

30g tomato purée
1 tsp garlic powder
1 tsp water
85g reduced-fat mozzarella, grated
5 cherry tomatoes, sliced
Dried oregano, to serve

For the pizza base
85g self-raising flour
50g 0% fat Greek yogurt

1. Preheat the oven to 190°C.
2. To make the pizza dough, put 55g of the flour and the Greek yogurt in a large bowl and mix thoroughly with a wooden spoon until the mixture forms a ball.
3. Dust a clean surface with 20g flour. Turn the dough ball out onto the floured surface and use your hands to flatten, squeeze and shape, turning over to ensure the dough doesn't stick to the surface by using all the flour. Roll out with a rolling pin until you have a 25cm pizza base. This part will take 5–10 minutes.
4. Scatter the remaining 10g flour over a baking sheet and carefully transfer the pizza base on to the sheet.
5. Mix the tomato purée, garlic powder and water together in a small bowl, then spread evenly across the pizza base.
6. Scatter over the grated mozzarella and top with the cherry tomatoes.
7. Bake for 6–8 minutes until the cheese has melted and the base is golden and crispy. Sprinkle some dried oregano over the top and serve.

PEPPERONI PIZZA

A pepperoni pizza is often seen as off-limits for anyone trying to reduce their calories to lose weight, but just swapping a few simple ingredients means you can enjoy this meat feast for a whopping 409 calories less than a supermarket version.

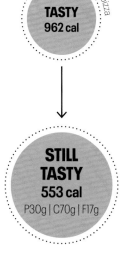

TASTY
962 cal
supermarket pizza

STILL TASTY
553 cal
P30g | C70g | F17g

TAKES 25 minutes

30g tomato purée
1 tsp water
50g reduced-fat mozzarella
¼ green pepper, sliced
A few fresh rocket leaves
30g pepperoni slices
Black pepper

For the pizza base
85g self-raising flour
50g 0% fat Greek yogurt

1. Preheat the oven to 190°C.
2. Put 55g of the flour and the Greek yogurt in a large bowl and mix thoroughly with a wooden spoon until the mixture forms a ball.
3. Dust a clean surface with 20g flour. Turn the dough ball out onto the floured surface and use your hands to flatten, squeeze and shape, turning over to ensure the dough doesn't stick to the surface by using all the flour. Roll out with a rolling pin until you have a 25cm pizza base. This part will take 5–10 minutes.
4. Scatter the remaining 10g flour over a baking sheet and carefully transfer the pizza base on to the sheet.
5. Mix the tomato purée and water together in a small bowl, then spread evenly over the pizza base.
6. Scatter over the mozzarella, pepper, rocket and pepperoni.
7. Bake for 12–15 minutes until the cheese has melted and base is crispy and golden. Add a twist of black pepper and serve.

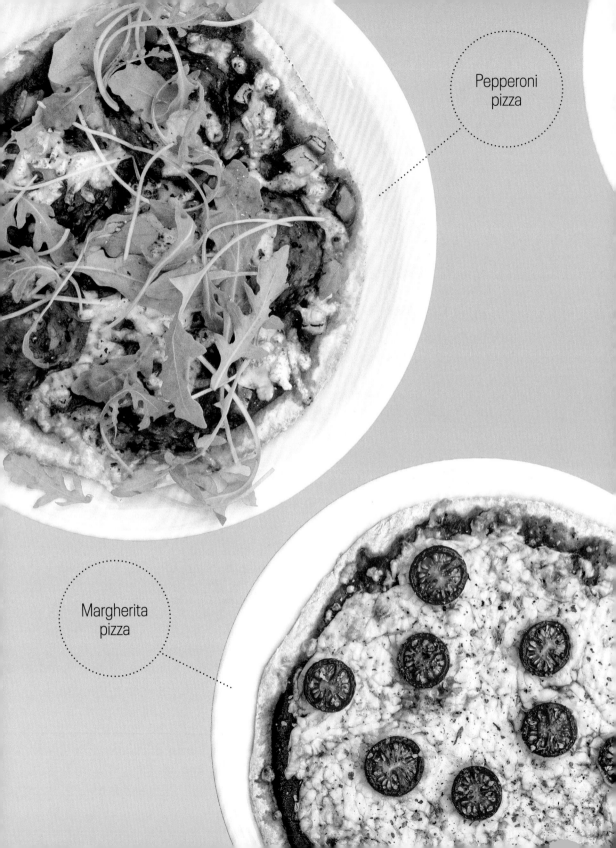

Pepperoni
pizza

Margherita
pizza

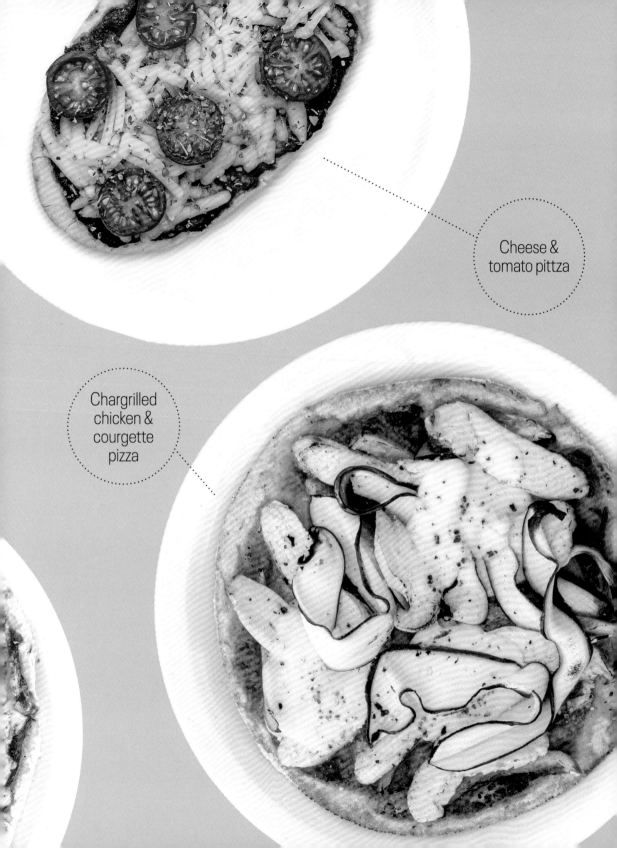

Cheese &
tomato pittza

Chargrilled
chicken &
courgette
pizza

CHARGRILLED CHICKEN
& COURGETTE PIZZA

By making your own pizza base with flour and 0% fat Greek yogurt, swapping 100g mozzarella for 50g fresh, light mozzarella and leaving out the olive oil often drizzled over to serve, you can save 268 calories and still enjoy a great-tasting pizza.

TAKES 25 minutes

30g tomato purée
1 tsp water
10g courgette
50g light mozzarella, sliced
75g cooked skinless chicken breast, sliced into 4cm pieces
¼ green pepper, sliced
Small handful of basil leaves
Black pepper

For the pizza base
85g self-raising flour
50g 0% fat Greek yogurt

1. Preheat the oven to 190°C.
2. Put 55g of the flour and the Greek yogurt in a large bowl and mix thoroughly with a wooden spoon until the mixture forms a ball.
3. Turn the dough ball out onto the floured surface and use your hands to flatten, squeeze and shape, turning over to ensure the dough doesn't stick to the surface by using all the flour. Roll out with a rolling pin until you have a 25cm pizza base. This part will take 5–10 minutes.
4. Scatter the remaining 10g flour over a baking sheet and carefully transfer the pizza base on to the sheet.
5. Mix the tomato purée and water together in a small bowl, then spread evenly across the tortilla.
6. Use a potato peeler to add thin slices of courgette, then scatter over the mozzarella, chicken, pepper and basil leaves.
7. Bake for 10–12 minutes until the cheese has melted and the base is crispy and golden. Finish with a twist of black pepper and serve.

CHEESE & TOMATO
PITTZA

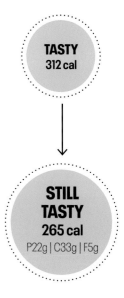

TASTY
312 cal

STILL TASTY
265 cal
P22g | C33g | F5g

If you fancy a quick, snack-sized portion of pizza, look no further than this easy pizza pitta bread. By swapping out the mozzarella for the same amount of a reduced-fat version, you can save 47 calories. If you enjoy two of these a week for a year, that's a saving of nearly 5,000 calories with hardly any effort.

TAKES 10 minutes

20g tomato purée
1 tsp water
1 tsp dried basil
1 pitta bread

40g reduced-fat mozzarella, grated
3 cherry tomatoes, chopped
1 tsp dried oregano

1. Preheat the oven to 175°C.
2. Mix the tomato purée, water and dried basil together in a small bowl, then spread evenly across the pitta bread.
3. Transfer to a small, foil-lined baking dish and scatter over the mozzarella and cherry tomatoes.
4. Bake for 5 minutes until the cheese has melted. Garnish with the dried oregano and serve.

HAM & PINEAPPLE
TORTILLA PIZZA

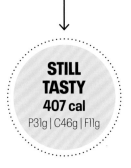

TASTY
684 cal

STILL TASTY
407 cal
P31g | C46g | F11g

By switching out the regular pizza base for a tortilla wrap, reducing the mozzarella from 100g to 30g and swapping it for a reduced-fat variety, you save 277 calories and can still tuck into your favourite American-style pizza. Italians look away now...

TAKES 10 minutes

20g tomato purée
1 tsp water
1 large tortilla wrap
75g cooked ham slices
50g pineapple chunks, finely chopped

30g reduced-fat mozzarella, grated
1 tsp dried oregano
Small handful of fresh rocket

1. Preheat the oven to 200°C.
2. Mix the tomato purée and water together in a small bowl, then sp read evenly across the tortilla wrap.
3. Scatter over the ham, pineapple, mozzarella, oregano and rocket.
4. Bake for 6–8 minutes until the cheese has melted and the tortilla is golden. Serve.

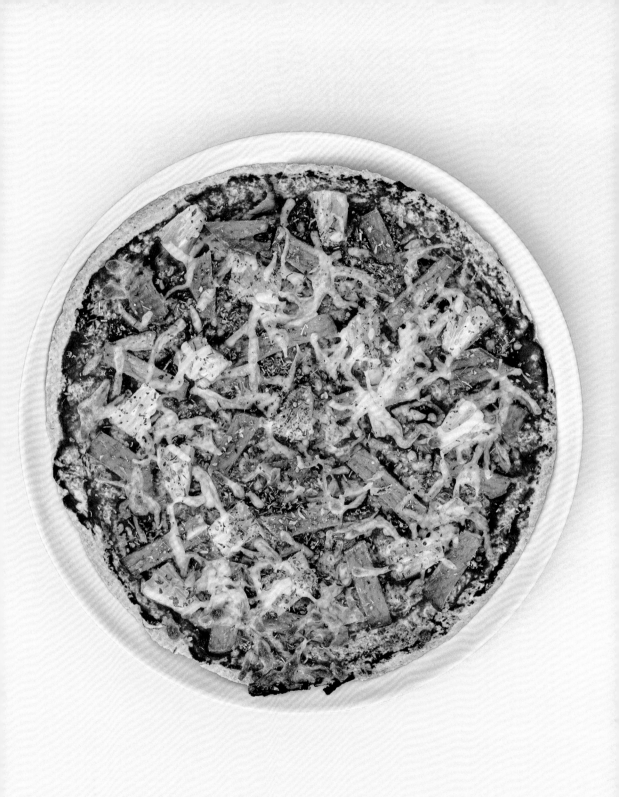

FETA & CARAMELIZED ONION
TORTILLA PIZZA

TASTY
478 cal

STILL TASTY
363 cal
P12g | C45g | F15g

Swap a large supermarket pizza base for a large tortilla wrap and reduce the usual 10ml olive oil to 2ml and pizza can still be on the menu for dinner. And you save 115 calories.

TAKES 15 minutes

2ml olive oil
¼ small onion, finely chopped
5g light soft brown sugar
15ml balsamic vinegar
20g tomato purée
1 tsp water

1 tsp dried basil
1 large tortilla wrap
50g feta cheese, crumbled
Small handful of baby spinach
1 tsp dried oregano

1. Put a small saucepan over a medium heat, add the olive oil, onion, brown sugar and balsamic vinegar and fry for 3–5 minutes, stirring regularly until it bubbles and thickens.
2. Meanwhile, preheat the oven to 200°C.
3. Mix the tomato purée, water and basil together in a small bowl, then spread evenly across the tortilla wrap.
4. Scatter the caramelized onions over the tortilla and top with the crumbled feta and spinach.
5. Bake for 5 minutes, or 7–8 minutes if you like the base extra crispy.
6. Scatter the dried oregano on top and serve.

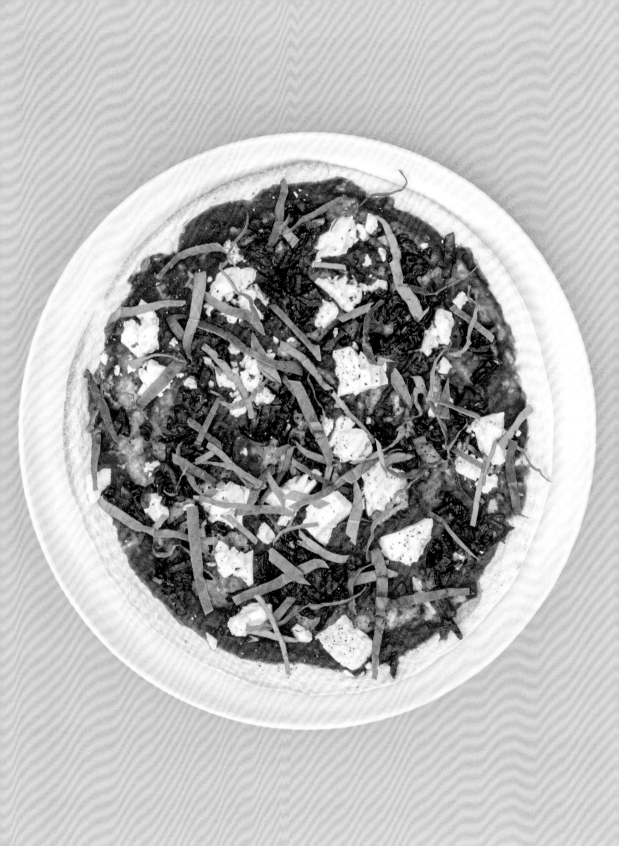

PARMA HAM
TORTILLA CALZONE

You can still tuck into a calzone pizza and lose weight! Simply swap the traditional pizza base for a large tortilla wrap, switch the mozzarella for a reduced-fat version and ditch the 10ml olive oil to save 271 calories.

TAKES 15 minutes

100ml passata
1 garlic clove, crushed
3 medium button mushrooms, finely sliced
1 large tortilla wrap
50g Parma ham slices
50g reduced-fat mozzarella, grated
Small handful of fresh rocket
Black pepper

1. Put a small saucepan over a high heat, then add the passata, garlic, sliced mushrooms and a twist of black pepper and bring to the boil. Cook for about 5 minutes until it has reduced to a thick sauce.
2. Preheat the oven to 200°C.
3. Put the tortilla wrap in a foil-lined, shallow baking dish. Spread the tomato sauce evenly over the tortilla and scatter over the Parma ham slices, mozzarella and rocket. Carefully fold the tortilla in half, trying not to spill any toppings.
4. Bake for 5–7 minutes until the tortilla is golden on top and the cheese has melted. Serve with a twist of black pepper.

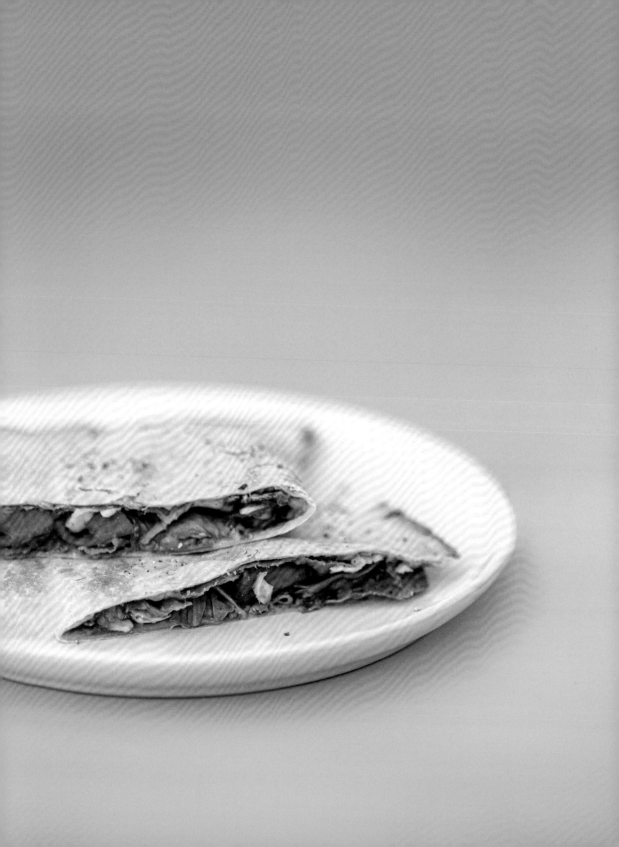

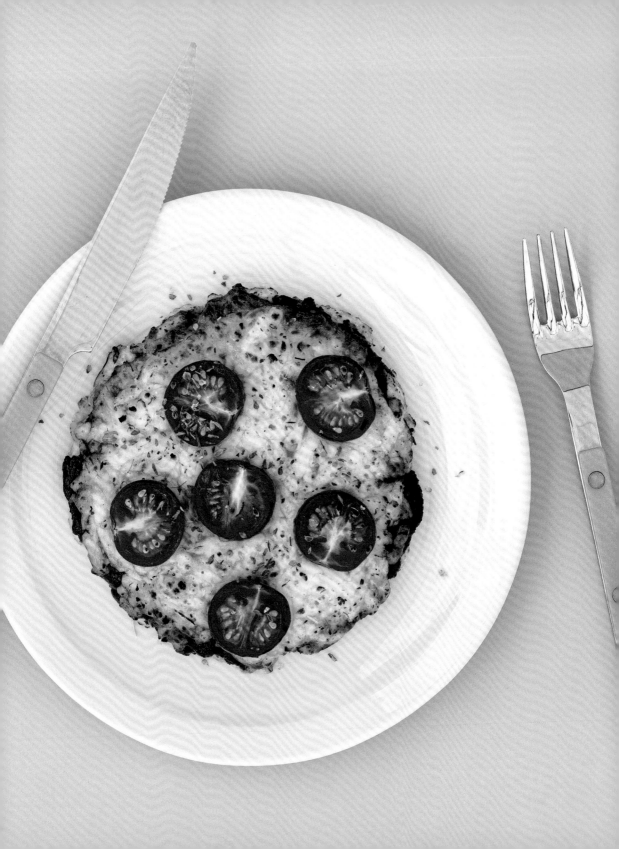

CHEESE & TOMATO
MEATZA

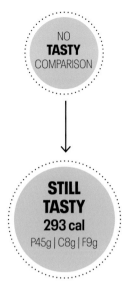

This alternative pizza recipe uses meat for the base instead of the usual dough, so you get a big portion of protein and your favourite pizza toppings, but you'll be eating significantly fewer calories than a regular pizza.

TAKES 20 minutes

125g turkey breast mince
½ tsp salt
½ tsp black pepper
A few basil leaves, chopped
10 × sprays olive oil cooking spray

30g tomato purée
50g light Mozzarella, grated
3 cherry tomatoes, sliced
A few baby spinach leaves
½ tsp dried oregano

1. Preheat the grill to high.
2. Put the turkey mince, salt, black pepper and chopped basil in a large mixing bowl and mix thoroughly with your hands until evenly combined. Then form into a large meatball and press down until you have an 15–20cm meat pizza base 1–2cm thick.
3. Spray a medium frying pan with the oil and set over a medium heat. Carefully add the meat base and cook for 2 minutes on each side to seal.
4. Grill the base for 5 minutes each side until it is slightly golden. Then spread the tomato purée evenly over the meat base and scatter over the mozzarella and cherry tomatoes.
5. Grill for a further 5 minutes until the mozzarella has melted and the base is golden brown. Garnish with the dried oregano and serve.

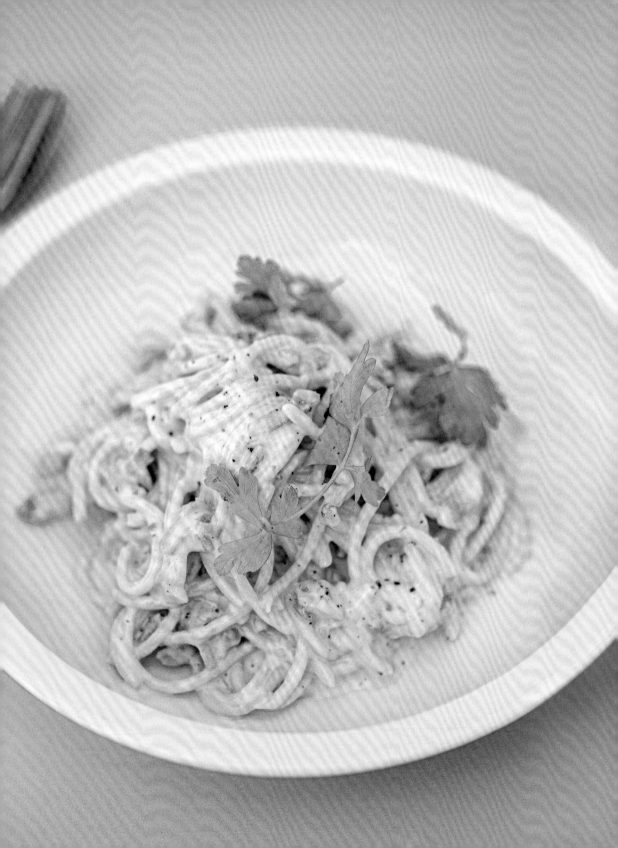

SPAGHETTI CARBONARA

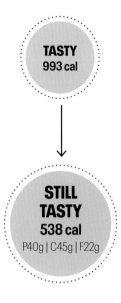

TASTY
993 cal

STILL TASTY
538 cal
P40g | C45g | F22g

This dish is undoubtedly a classic, but if you want to lose weight it's probably not a meal you enjoy regularly. However, by switching the bacon rashers for bacon medallions, soft cheese for a 50% reduced-fat version, whole milk for semi-skimmed, normal Cheddar for 50% reduced-fat, 10ml olive oil for 5ml and ditching the butter, you can nearly halve the calories. The trademark carbonara taste but with a huge saving of 455 calories.

TAKES 15 minutes

50g uncooked spaghetti
5ml olive oil
3 bacon medallions, chopped
4 spring onions, chopped
1 medium egg

75g 50% reduced-fat soft cheese
75ml semi-skimmed milk
25g 50% reduced-fat Cheddar
  cheese, grated
Black pepper

1. Fill a large saucepan with water and bring to the boil. Break the spaghetti in half and add to pan. Cook for 6–8 minutes until soft and tender.
2. While the spaghetti is cooking, put a medium pan over a medium heat and add the olive oil and bacon. Cook for 5 minutes, stirring with spatula, until the bacon begins to brown.
3. Crack the egg into a medium bowl, add the soft cheese and whisk with a fork until evenly combined.
4. Gradually add the milk and grated Cheddar and stir for 3–5 minutes until the cheese has melted and the sauce has thickened slightly. Then add the spring onions.
5. Pour the sauce into the pan over the bacon and cook over a low heat for 1 minute, stirring constantly.
6. Take the pan off the heat, drain the spaghetti, then add to the pan to stir into the carbonara sauce. Serve with a twist of black pepper.

SPICY RED PESTO
CHICKEN PASTA

Here's an equally delicious red pesto pasta variation with a kick, plus added chicken to increase your protein. This recipe uses reduced-fat red pesto and 15 sprays of cooking oil to save 149 calories.

TAKES 15 minutes

20 × sprays olive oil cooking spray
10g garlic paste
150g skinless chicken breast, cut into 4cm pieces
50g uncooked fusilli
5g pine nuts
40g reduced-fat red pesto

½ red pepper, finely chopped
10 green beans, halved
Small bunch of fresh flat-leaf parsley, chopped
1 red chilli, deseeded and finely chopped
Salt and pepper

1. Spray a medium pan with the oil and set over a medium heat. Add the garlic paste and chicken and cook for 5 minutes, turning regularly with a spatula.
2. While the chicken is cooking, fill a small saucepan with water and bring to the boil. Add the pasta and simmer for 6–8 minutes until tender. Drain and set aside.
3. Add the drained pasta, pine nuts, red pesto, red pepper, green beans and parsley to the chicken, reduce the heat and stir thoroughly. Cook over a low heat for 6–8 minutes, adding a little water if it starts to dry out too much.
4. Lastly, add the chilli and mix through. Season with salt and pepper to taste before serving.

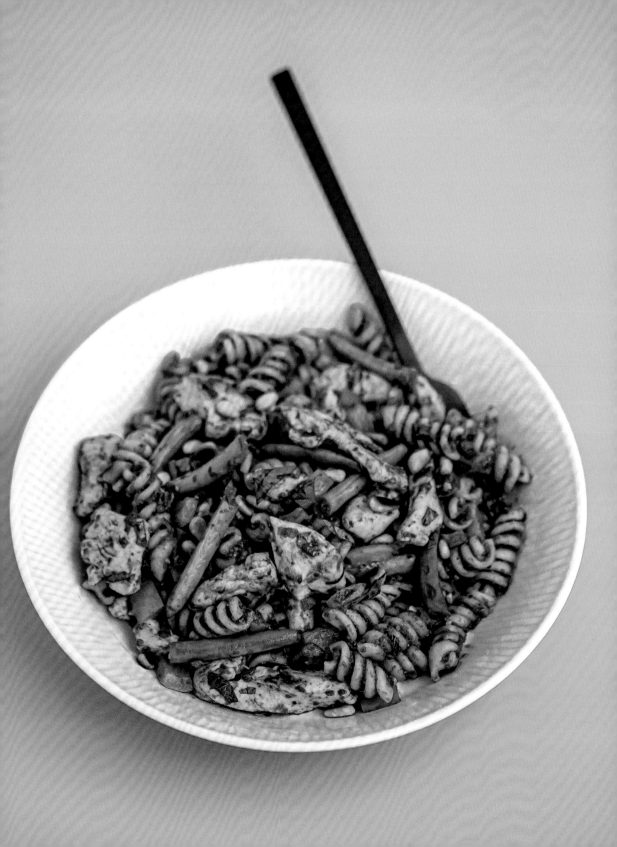

CHEESY
GREEN PESTO PASTA

Many people think that they can't eat pasta and lose weight, but there's simply no evidence to support this. In fact, you can definitely have pasta when trying to slim down and you can even enjoy it with cheese and pesto, too. The key is understanding portion sizes and finding the perfect balance of taste and calories. Here we are swapping the pesto and Cheddar for reduced-fat versions and leaving out the 10ml olive oil many people add to the pan. Same portion, same great taste, but 316 fewer calories.

TAKES 15 minutes

75g uncooked penne
½ red onion, finely chopped
½ yellow pepper, finely chopped
1 garlic clove, crushed
5 sun-dried tomatoes, finely chopped
¼ medium aubergine, finely chopped

Small handful of freshly chopped basil
40g reduced-fat green pesto
1 tsp dried oregano
50g reduced-fat Cheddar cheese, grated
Salt and pepper

1. Fill a medium saucepan with water and bring to the boil. Add the pasta and cook for 6–8 minutes until tender. Drain and set aside.
2. While the pasta is cooking, add the red onion, pepper, garlic, sun-dried tomatoes, aubergine and basil to a medium frying pan with the green pesto. Cook over a low heat for 5 minutes.
3. Add the drained pasta, mix thoroughly and season with the dried oregano and salt and pepper.
4. Finally, plate up the pesto pasta, sprinkle over the cheese and allow it to melt in. To melt faster, microwave the dish on full power for 20 seconds. Serve.

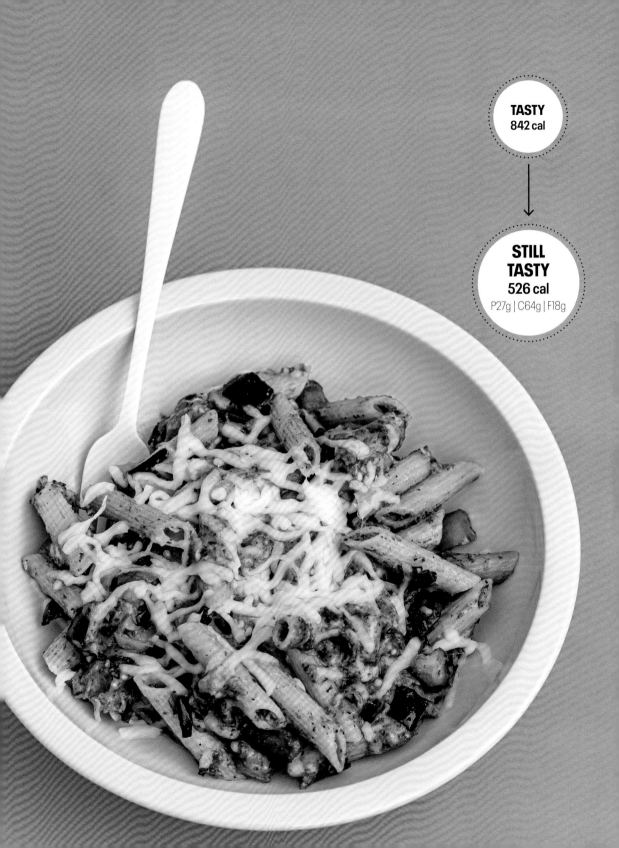

TASTY
842 cal

STILL TASTY
526 cal
P27g | C64g | F18g

SPINACH & RICOTTA
TAGLIATELLE

By simply reducing the usual 20g butter to 10g in this recipe, you can save 75 calories while still enjoying the same-sized portion and flavours of a classic spinach and ricotta pasta.

TAKES 15 minutes

75g uncooked tagliatelle
75g spinach, chopped
10g unsalted butter
1 garlic clove, crushed

5g pine nuts
50g ricotta cheese
Salt and pepper

1. Half-fill a medium saucepan with water and bring to the boil. Add the tagliatelle and simmer for 6–8 minutes until tender. Drain and set aside.
2. While the pasta is cooking, add a drop of water to a medium pan, set over a medium-high heat and add the spinach. Stir for 1–2 minutes until wilted, then drain through a sieve, squeezing out as much water as possible.
3. Return the spinach to the pan over a medium-low heat, then add the butter, garlic, pine nuts and ricotta and mix with a wooden spoon for 2 minutes. Add more pasta cooking water if it becomes too dry.
4. Add the drained tagliatelle and mix in thoroughly for 2 minutes. Season with salt and pepper to taste and serve.

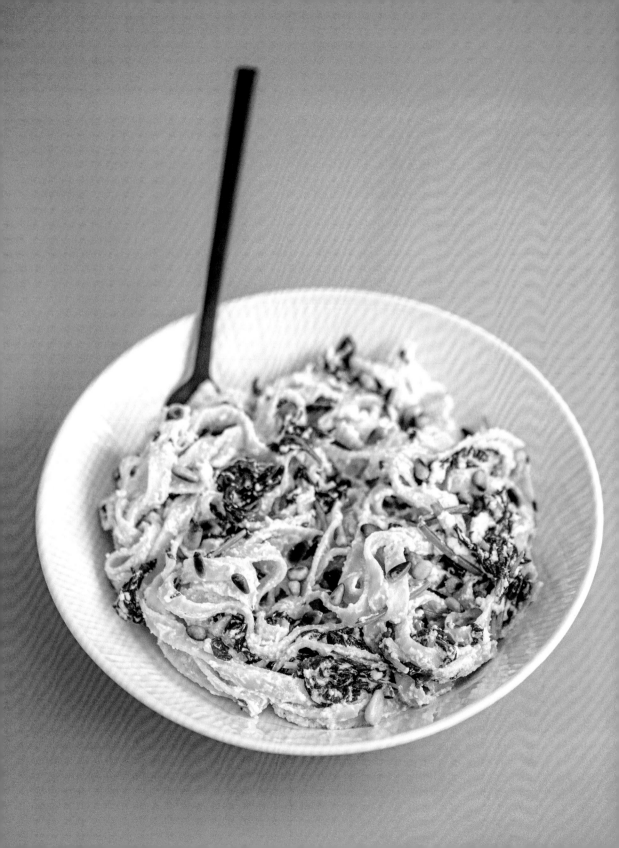

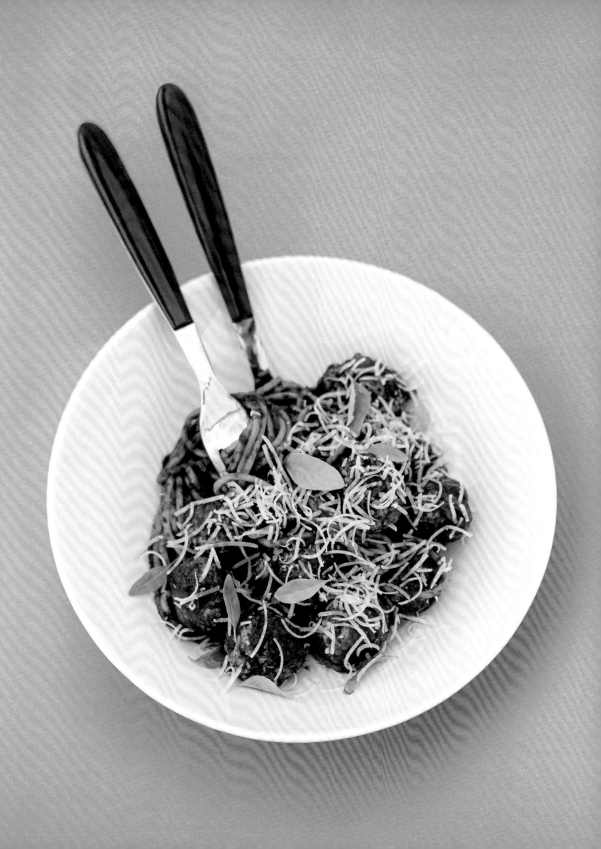

SPAGHETTI
MEATBALLS

TASTY
927 cal

STILL TASTY
604 cal
P54g | C70g | F12g

Switch 20% fat pork mince for 5% fat, swap 10ml olive oil for 10 sprays of olive oil cooking spray, halve the Parmesan from 10g to 5g and you can save 323 calories to support you on your way to achieving your weight-loss goal.

TAKES 20 minutes

10 × sprays olive oil cooking spray
75g uncooked spaghetti
150g passata
20g tomato purée
Small handful of fresh basil leaves
1 tsp dried oregano
5g Parmesan cheese, grated
Salt
Squeeze of lemon juice

For the meatballs
150g 5% fat pork mince
5ml olive oil
¼ red onion, finely chopped
1 tsp garlic powder
½ tsp black pepper

1. Put all the meatball ingredients in a large mixing bowl and mix together with your hands until evenly combined. Then form the mixture into 6 small meatballs.
2. Spray a saucepan with the oil, set over a medium heat and tilt the pan until the base of the pan is covered with the oil. Add the meatballs and sear for 3–4 minutes. Reduce the heat and cook for a further 5 minutes.
3. Fill a large saucepan with water, bring to the boil and add the spaghetti. Cook for 6–8 minutes until tender, then drain and set aside.
4. Add the passata, tomato purée, basil, oregano and a pinch of salt to the meatballs and simmer for 10 minutes, stirring regularly.
5. Add the drained spaghetti to the meatballs and stir until the pasta is covered in tomato sauce. Then stir in the lemon juice briefly.
6. Serve with the grated Parmesan sprinkled over the top and fresh basil leaves, if you wish.

MAC 'N CHEESE

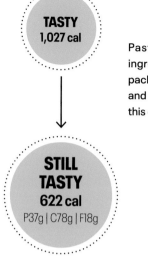

TASTY
1,027 cal

STILL
TASTY
622 cal
P37g | C78g | F18g

Pasta, butter and cheese are some of the most calorific ingredients, so when combined they naturally produce a meal packed full of calories. But by reducing the butter from 15g to 5g and using only 75g 50% reduced-fat Cheddar, you can still enjoy this comfort food classic AND save a whopping 405 calories!

TAKES 30 minutes

60g uncooked macaroni
5g unsalted butter
½ onion, finely chopped
25g plain flour
125ml semi-skimmed milk

75g 50% reduced-fat Cheddar cheese, grated
10g dried breadcrumbs
Black pepper

1. Half-fill a small saucepan with water, bring to the boil, then add the macaroni. Cook for 6–8 minutes until tender. Drain and set aside.
2. Preheat the oven to 200°C.
3. While the macaroni is cooking, put a medium saucepan over a low heat and add the butter, onion and flour. Stir with a wooden spoon for 2–3 minutes, then add the milk and 50g of the cheese.
4. Add the drained macaroni to the cheese sauce and stir thoroughly, then transfer the pasta to a 12 × 16cm ovenproof baking dish. Top the macaroni with the remaining cheese, the breadcrumbs and some black pepper.
5. Bake for 20 minutes until golden and bubbling. Serve.

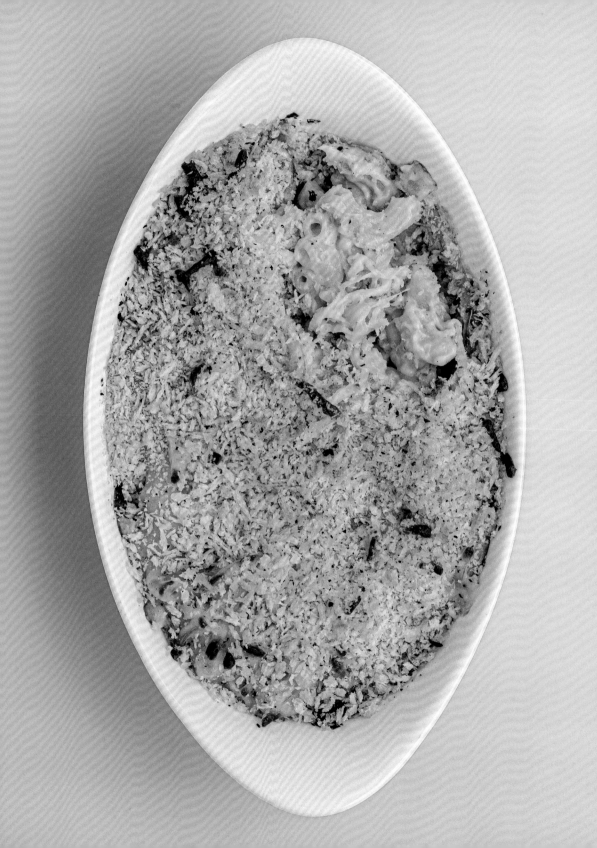

SEA BASS
LINGUINE

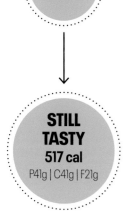

TASTY
687 cal

STILL TASTY
517 cal

P41g | C41g | F21g

A white fish dish is often regarded as good for weight loss as it's generally low in calories. But despite this, when you're out in a restaurant there's a good chance that the sauce will include a large amount of butter or additional oil. As sea bass already contains a moderate amount of fish oil, simply removing 10ml olive oil, choosing to bake instead of fry the fish, and reducing the butter from 10g to 5g, means you get a tasty fish pasta and a saving of 170 calories.

TAKES 20 minutes

150g sea bass fillets, skin on
5g unsalted butter
1 tbsp white wine
4 cherry tomatoes, chopped
Juice of 1 lemon
2 garlic cloves, crushed
50g uncooked linguine
15g baby capers, drained and finely chopped

Small handful of freshly chopped flat-leaf parsley
50g 0% fat Greek yogurt
Salt and pepper
Small handful of freshly chopped coriander

1. Preheat the oven to 200°C.
2. Put the sea bass fillets in the centre of a large piece of kitchen foil, spread the butter evenly over each fillet and top with the white wine, cherry tomatoes, lemon juice, garlic, ½ teaspoon of salt and ½ teaspoon of pepper. Tightly close up the foil and transfer to a large baking tray. Bake for 15 minutes.
3. While the sea bass is cooking, half-fill a medium saucepan with water and bring to the boil. Add the linguine and cook for 6–8 minutes until tender. Drain, return to the pan and set aside.
4. To make the pasta sauce, combine the capers, parsley and Greek yogurt with some salt and pepper.
5. Carefully unwrap the foil parcel, then remove the skin from the sea bass fillets with a knife and fork and discard. Cut the sea bass into small chunks and add to the saucepan with the drained linguine along with the butter and vegetables in the foil. Stir in thoroughly.
6. Add the pasta sauce and coriander to the sea bass and linguine and warm over a low heat for 1 minute. Serve.

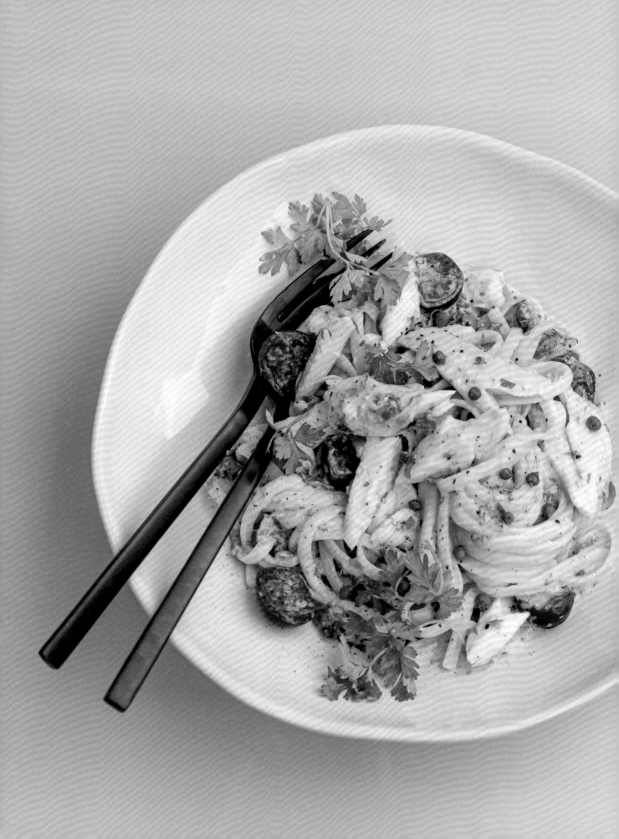

TUNA & SWEETCORN
PASTA BAKE

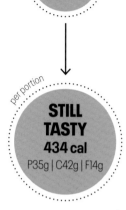

TASTY
537 cal

per portion

STILL TASTY
434 cal
P35g | C42g | F14g

The sauce is often the most calorie-dense part of pasta dishes. But if you make the cheese sauce for a pasta bake with 10g butter rather than the usual 50g, skimmed instead of whole milk and 50% reduced-fat Cheddar, you can still eat the same amount, enjoy the same flavours AND save 103 calories per portion.

TAKES 25 minutes
MAKES 4 portions

250g uncooked penne or fusilli
10g unsalted butter
30g plain flour
300ml skimmed milk
150g 50% reduced-fat Cheddar cheese, grated
2 × 120g tins of tuna, drained

200g tinned sweetcorn, drained
2 spring onions, finely sliced
1 tbsp dried Italian herbs
1 large tomato, sliced
Salt and pepper
Small handful of fresh chopped parsley

1. Preheat the oven to 200°C.
2. Fill a large saucepan with water, bring to the boil and add the pasta. Cook for 6–8 minutes.
3. While the pasta is cooking, put a small saucepan over a low heat and add the butter, flour and milk. Slowly combine with a wooden spoon before adding half of the grated cheese. Stir for 4–5 minutes until the sauce thickens.
4. Drain the pasta, return to the saucepan, then add the cheese sauce and slowly mix in with a wooden spoon, along with the tuna, sweetcorn, spring onions, Italian herbs and some salt and pepper. Transfer to a large, ovenproof baking dish.
5. Top with the remaining cheese and the tomato slices and bake for 10–15 minutes until golden and crispy. Serve with fresh parsley scattered over the top.

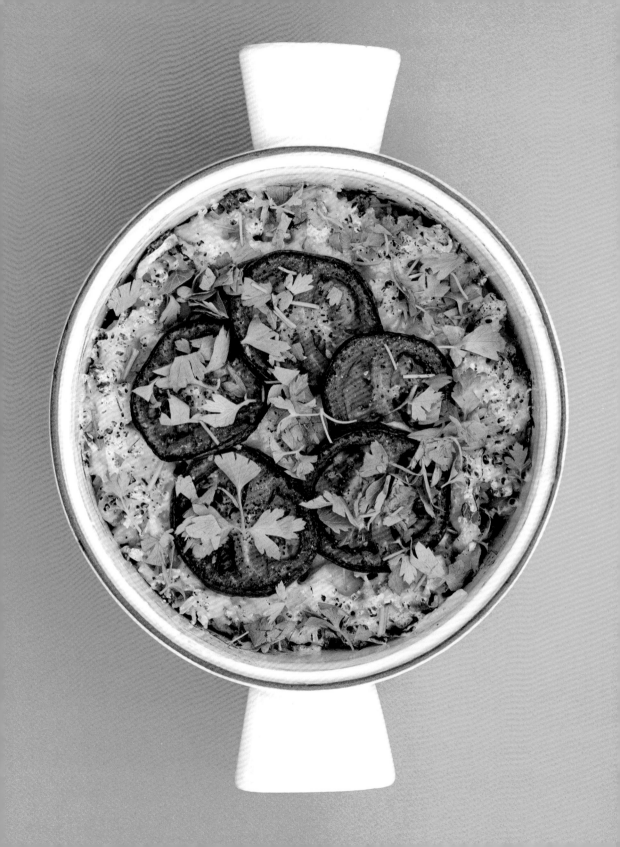

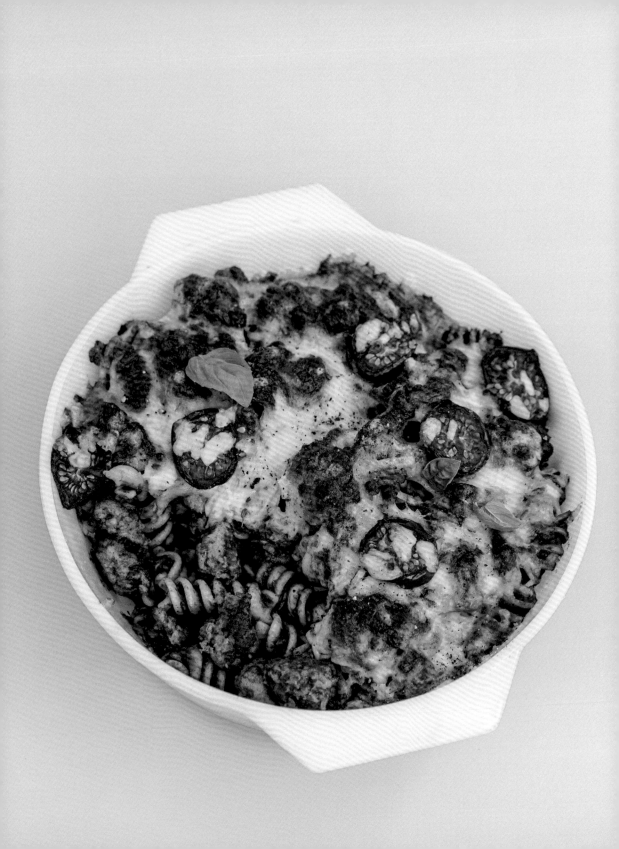

SAUSAGE & TOMATO
PASTA BAKE

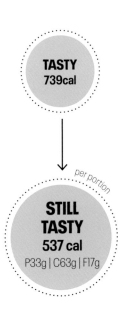

TASTY
739cal

per portion

STILL
TASTY
537 cal
P33g | C63g | F17g

By switching regular pork sausages for a low-fat option, swapping 10ml olive oil for 10 sprays of cooking oil and using 50% reduced-fat Cheddar you still get a delicious pasta bake, but for 202 fewer calories per portion.

TAKES 25 minutes
MAKES 4 portions

10 × sprays garlic oil cooking spray
6 reduced-fat pork sausages, cut into 2cm slices
1 onion, finely sliced
250g uncooked penne or fusilli
10g unsalted butter
5g fennel seeds
1 tsp garlic purée

30g tomato purée
30g plain flour
500g passata
1 tbsp dried Italian herbs
150g 50% reduced-fat Cheddar cheese, grated
10 cherry tomatoes, chopped
Salt and pepper

1. Preheat the oven to 200°C.
2. Spray a large saucepan with the oil, set over a medium heat and add the sausages and onion. Cook for 7–8 minutes, using a spatula to turn the sausages regularly.
3. Fill a large saucepan with water, bring to the boil and add the pasta. Cook for 6–8 minutes.
4. While the pasta is cooking, put a small saucepan over a low heat and add the butter, fennel seeds, garlic purée, tomato purée, flour and passata. Slowly combine with a wooden spoon for 4–5 minutes until the sauce thickens.
5. Drain the pasta and return it to the pan, then add the tomato sauce, sausages and onion, Italian herbs and some salt and pepper. Mix with a wooden spoon until the pasta is evenly covered. Transfer to a large, ovenproof baking dish.
6. Top with the cheese and chopped cherry tomatoes and bake for 10–15 minutes until golden and crispy. Serve.

LASAGNE

Lasagne is one of the all-time most popular dishes the world over. But if you order it in a restaurant or follow your favourite chef's recipe, it will be packed with calories. A few simple swaps and you can enjoy it AND lose weight, meaning it can be on your menu more often. Switch the 20% fat beef mince for 5% fat, 10ml olive oil for 5ml, forego the cheese sauce for half-fat crème fraîche and swap the mozzarella for a reduced-fat variety for great-tasting lasagne and a massive saving of 436 calories. Buon appetito!

TAKES 35 minutes

3 dried lasagne sheets (80g)	100g passata
5ml olive oil	5 cherry tomatoes, chopped
100g 5% fat beef mince	30g half-fat crème fraîche
2 garlic cloves, crushed	100g reduced-fat mozzarella, grated
½ onion, finely chopped	Salt and pepper

1. Preheat the oven to 200°C.
2. Put the lasagne sheets in a large bowl or cooking tray full of warm water and leave to soak for 10 minutes.
3. While the lasagne sheets are softening, set a large saucepan over a medium heat. Add the olive oil, beef mince, garlic and onion and cook for 2–3 minutes until the mince begins to brown. Then add the passata and chopped cherry tomatoes, season with salt and pepper and stir with a spatula. Cook for a further 3 minutes.
4. Add one soaked lasagne sheet to the bottom of a lasagne dish or small roasting dish, then spoon one-third of the beef and sauce evenly on top followed by one-third of the crème fraîche and then one-third of the mozzarella. Repeat this twice more until you have used all the lasagne sheets, beef sauce and crème fraîche. Ensure all the lasagne sheets are covered with the beef sauce so that they soften.
5. Cook for 20–25 minutes. Then scatter over the remaining third of mozzarella and cook for a further 5 minutes until the cheese is melted and golden. Leave to cool for 5 minutes, then serve.

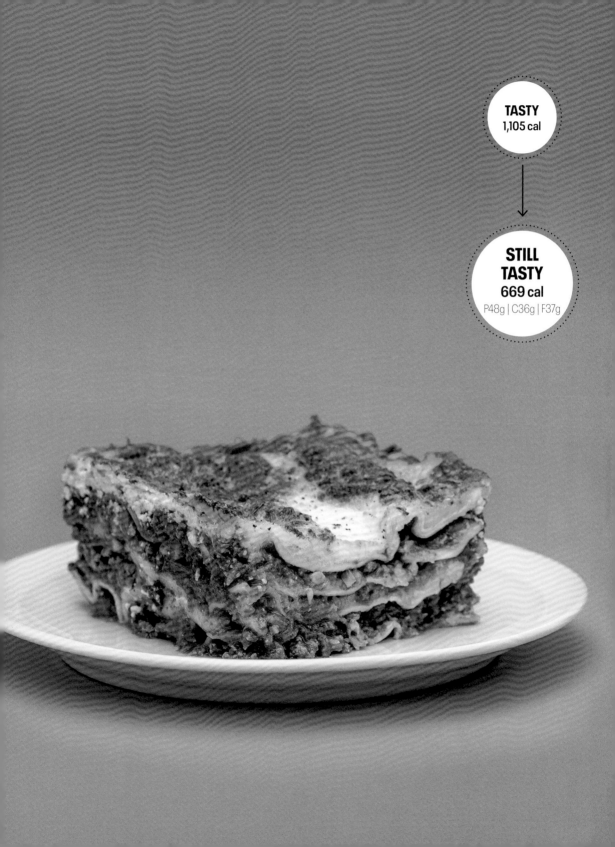

TASTY
1,105 cal

STILL
TASTY
669 cal
P48g | C36g | F37g

PAN-FRIED CHEESE
& CHORIZO GNOCCHI

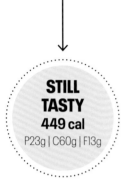

TASTY
555 cal

STILL TASTY
449 cal
P23g | C60g | F13g

Here's another delicious reduced-calorie Italian recipe. This super-speedy one-pan dish uses reduced-fat mozzarella and 5ml olive oil to save you 106 calories without sacrificing any of the flavour.

TAKES 10 minutes

5ml olive oil
150g gnocchi
150ml passata
20g chorizo slices
3 cherry tomatoes, chopped
Small handful of freshly chopped basil

1 tsp dried Italian herbs
50g reduced-fat mozzarella, grated
Black pepper

1. Put a medium saucepan over a medium heat and add the olive oil, then the gnocchi. Fry for 3–4 minutes until the gnocchi begins to brown.
2. Reduce the heat, then add the passata, chorizo, cherry tomatoes, basil and Italian herbs. Cook, stirring with a wooden spoon to ensure the gnocchi is covered in the sauce, for 3–4 minutes.
3. Transfer the gnocchi to an ovenproof serving dish, top with the grated mozzarella and allow it to melt. You can also microwave the dish on full power for 30 seconds to help the cheese melt quicker, if desired. Garnish with black pepper and serve with shredded basil if you wish.

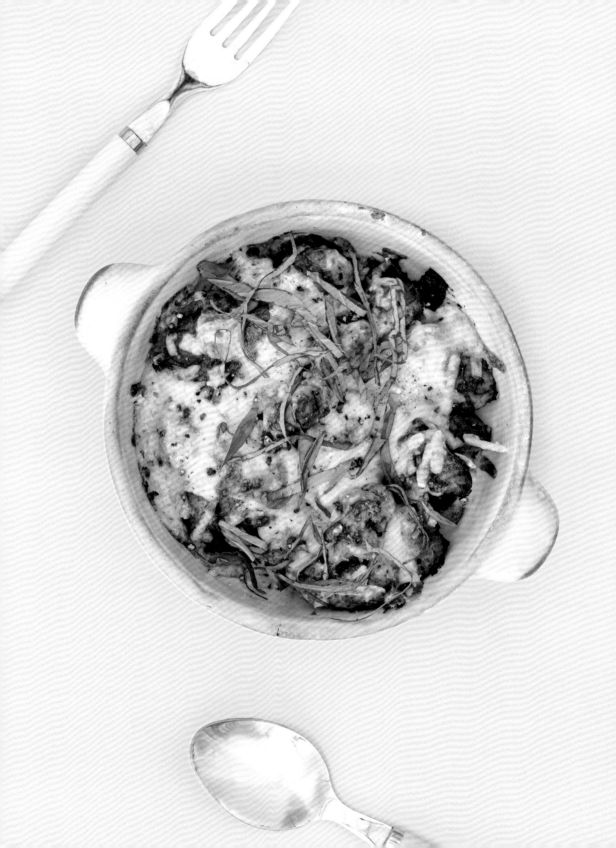

EASY CHICKEN, BACON
& MUSHROOM RISOTTO

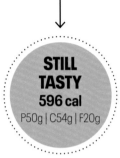

TASTY
890 cal

STILL
TASTY
596 cal
P50g | C54g | F20g

Many risotto recipes include big portions of butter, cooking oil and cheese. But reducing 15g butter to 5g, 75g Parmesan to 30g and 10ml olive oil to 5ml doesn't reduce the amount of hero ingredients, still provides loads of taste, and is 294 calories less than the original.

TAKES 35 minutes

5ml olive oil
100g skinless chicken breast,
 cut into 3cm pieces
2 bacon medallions, chopped
2 medium button mushrooms, sliced
1 garlic clove, crushed
½ onion, grated
60g risotto rice
250ml water

½ chicken stock cube
30g frozen peas
50ml white wine
5g unsalted butter
30g Parmesan cheese, grated
Small handful of freshly chopped
 flat-leaf parsley
Salt and pepper

1. Put a small saucepan over a medium heat and add the olive oil, chicken, bacon, mushrooms, garlic and grated onion. Cook for 5 minutes until the chicken and onion begin to brown.
2. Add the risotto rice, stir in briefly for 30 seconds before adding half the water and the stock cube. Stir until the stock cube dissolves.
3. Reduce the heat to low and simmer for 10 minutes, stirring often until the rice is soft and creamy.
4. Add the frozen peas, remaining water and the white wine, then stir for 2 minutes.
5. Stir in the butter and 20g of the Parmesan and cook until the butter melts. Add the parsley and season with salt and pepper. Scatter over the remaining Parmesan, stir in and serve.

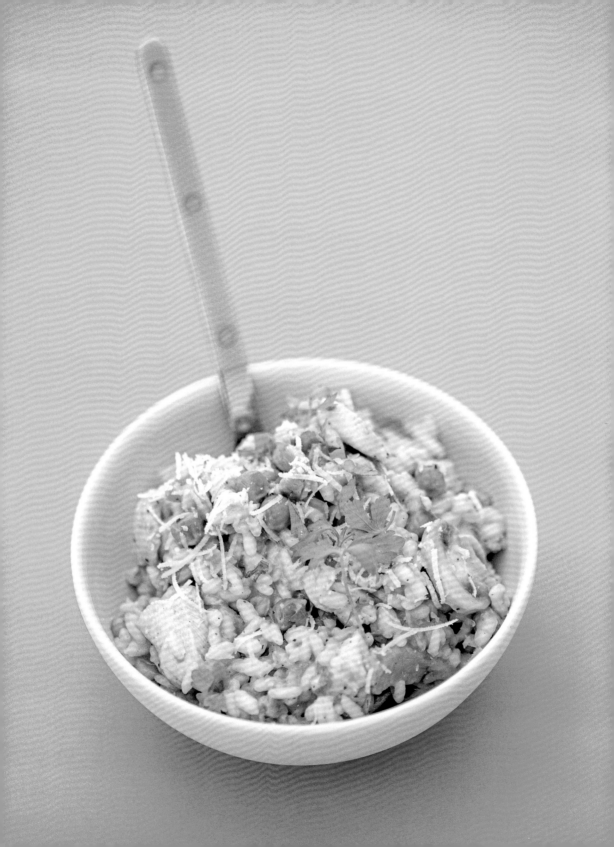

TEMPURA PRAWNS

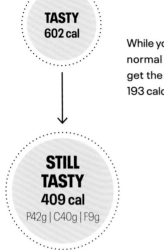

TASTY
602 cal

STILL TASTY
409 cal
P42g | C40g | F9g

While you can enjoy deep-fried foods in moderation, by swapping normal tempura prawns for this oven-baked version, you still get the crispy textures and sweet chilli dipping sauce but save 193 calories to support your weight-loss goal.

TAKES 30 minutes

1 medium egg

30g panko breadcrumbs

1 tsp garlic powder

½ tsp salt

10g plain flour

150g raw jumbo king prawns

10 × sprays olive oil cooking spray

30g sweet chilli sauce

1. Preheat the oven to 220°C.
2. Crack the egg into a medium bowl and whisk with a fork until smooth.
3. Put the panko breadcrumbs, garlic powder, salt and flour in a separate medium bowl and mix together with your hands.
4. Pat the prawns dry with three large pieces of kitchen paper. Dip the prawns in the beaten egg, then dip in the breadcrumb mixture to coat thoroughly.
5. Spray a clean oven shelf with the oil then place the tempura prawns on the shelf and put a baking tray underneath to catch any crumbs. Bake for 18–22 minutes, turning halfway through cooking.
6. Serve the tempura prawns with the sweet chilli sauce.

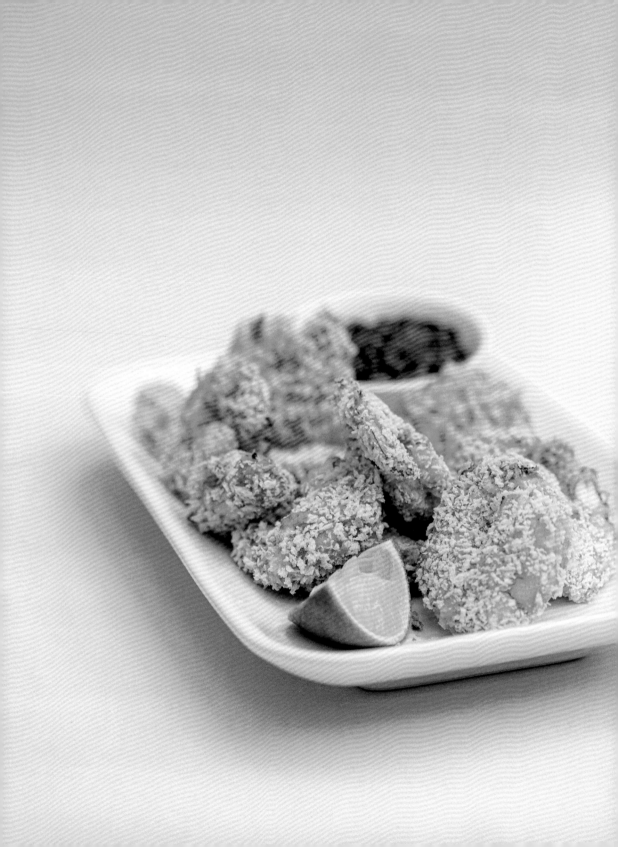

TERIYAKI SALMON
with potato rösti & broccoli

Salmon is rich in protein and omega-3 fats and it goes well with a variety of ingredients; here it accompanies potato rösti and Tenderstem broccoli. Average versions of this dish contain around 858 calories, but by switching up the fats and reducing the butter from 20g to 5g and swapping 15ml olive oil for 15 sprays of cooking oil you save yourself 189 calories.

TAKES 20 minutes

125g skinless salmon fillet
100g Tenderstem broccoli

For the teriyaki sauce
15ml light soy sauce
5g light soft brown sugar
1 tsp garlic powder
1cm piece of fresh ginger, peeled and grated
1 tsp white wine vinegar
1 tsp cornflour

For the potato rösti
200g new potatoes, peeled
¼ red onion, finely chopped
5g unsalted butter
25g plain flour
1 medium egg
15 × sprays butter-flavour cooking spray
Salt and pepper

To garnish
Small handful of freshly chopped coriander
¼ small red chilli, finely chopped
1 spring onion, sliced

1. Preheat the oven to 180°C.
2. To make the teriyaki sauce, put all the ingredients in a small bowl and mix thoroughly with a fork.
3. Put the salmon fillet on a foil-lined baking tray and carefully pour over the teriyaki sauce. Roast for 12–15 minutes, turning over halfway through cooking.
4. While the salmon is cooking, grate the potatoes on a cheese grater. With your hands, squeeze as much water out of the grated potatoes as possible and transfer to a medium bowl.
5. Add the red onion, butter and flour to the potatoes and season with salt and pepper. Then crack in the egg and mix all the ingredients together with a fork.

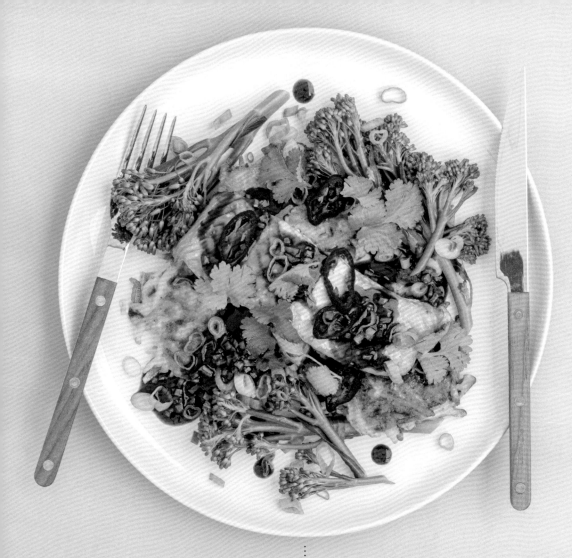

6. Spray a large frying pan with the cooking spray and set over a high heat. Add large tablespoons of the potato mixture and fry the rösti for 3–4 minutes on each side until crispy and golden brown. You should have 3–4 rösti in total.

7. While the rösti are frying, put the broccoli in a small saucepan and cover with water. Bring to the boil, reduce the heat and simmer for 3 minutes. Drain.

8. Plate up the teriyaki salmon with the potato rösti, broccoli, coriander, red chilli and spring onion. Serve.

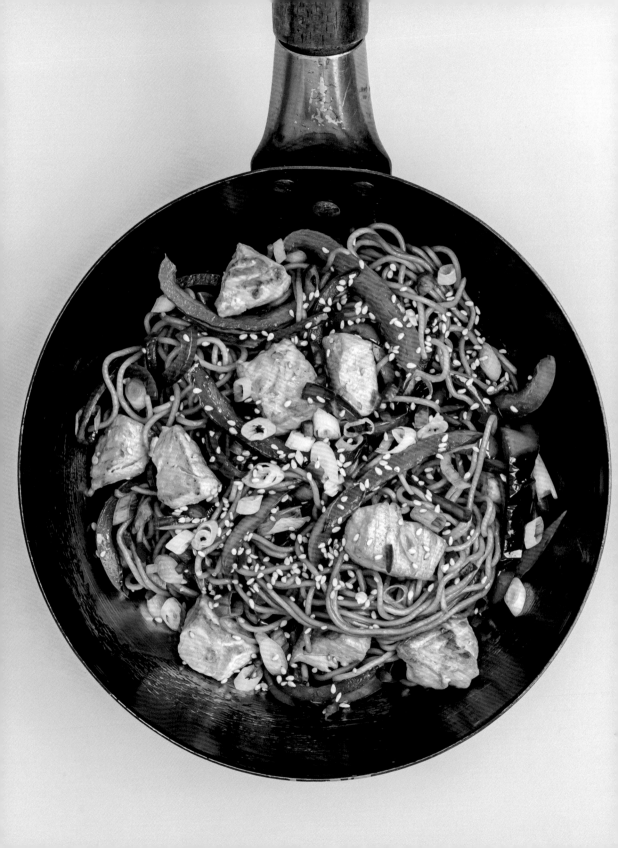

SALMON YAKI SOBA

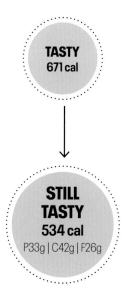

TASTY
671 cal

STILL TASTY
534 cal
P33g | C42g | F26g

Salmon yaki soba is a popular Japanese dish, but despite the fact it is rich in low-calorie vegetables and sauce, the amount of cooking oil can increase the calories. But fear not! Simply reduce the 20ml sesame oil to 5ml and you save 137 calories.

TAKES 15 minutes

125g salmon fillet	½ red pepper, sliced
Juice of ½ lime	½ green pepper, sliced
50g egg noodles	1 spring onion, finely chopped
5ml toasted sesame oil	¼ small red chilli, deseeded and
½ onion, sliced	finely chopped
1 tsp grated fresh ginger	1 tsp sesame seeds
10ml light soy sauce	Salt and pepper

1. Carefully remove the skin from the salmon by placing it on its side and slicing with a sharp kitchen knife. Then season with salt and black pepper and the lime juice.
2. Half-fill a small saucepan with water and bring to the boil. Add the noodles, reduce the heat and simmer for 4–6 minutes until tender. Drain.
3. While the noodles are cooking, put a medium wok or frying pan over a medium heat and add the sesame oil. Then add the onion, ginger, soy sauce, peppers and salmon. Cook for 4–6 minutes, stirring regularly. Don't worry if the salmon breaks apart.
4. Add the drained noodles, stir in thoroughly and cook for 2–3 minutes, adding a drop of water if it looks too dry.
5. Transfer to a serving dish and top with the chopped spring onion, red chilli and sesame seeds before serving.

CHICKEN YAKI SOBA

TASTY
728 cal

STILL
TASTY
436 cal
P40g | C42g | F12g

By swapping chicken thigh for chicken breast and reducing the sesame oil like we did in the Salmon Yaki Soba (see page 141), you can save 292 calories on this delicious noodle dish.

TAKES 15 minutes

50g egg noodles
5ml toasted sesame oil
125g skinless chicken breast, cut into 3cm pieces
½ onion, sliced
½ red pepper, sliced
½ green pepper, sliced
1 tsp grated fresh ginger
Juice of ½ lime

10ml light soy sauce
1 spring onion, finely sliced
5g salted peanuts, crushed
¼ small red chilli, deseeded and finely chopped
Small handful of freshly chopped coriander
Sprinkle of sesame seeds
Salt and pepper

1. Half-fill a small saucepan with water and bring to the boil. Add the noodles, reduce the heat and simmer for 4–6 minutes until tender. Drain.
2. While the noodles are cooking, put a medium wok or frying pan over a medium heat and add the sesame oil. Then add the chicken, onion, peppers, ginger, lime juice and soy sauce and season with salt and pepper. Cook for 6–8 minutes, stirring regularly.
3. Add the drained noodles, stir in thoroughly and cook for 2–3 minutes, adding a drop of water if it looks too dry.
4. Transfer to a serving dish and top with chopped spring onion, crushed peanuts, chilli, coriander and a sprinkling of sesame seeds before serving.

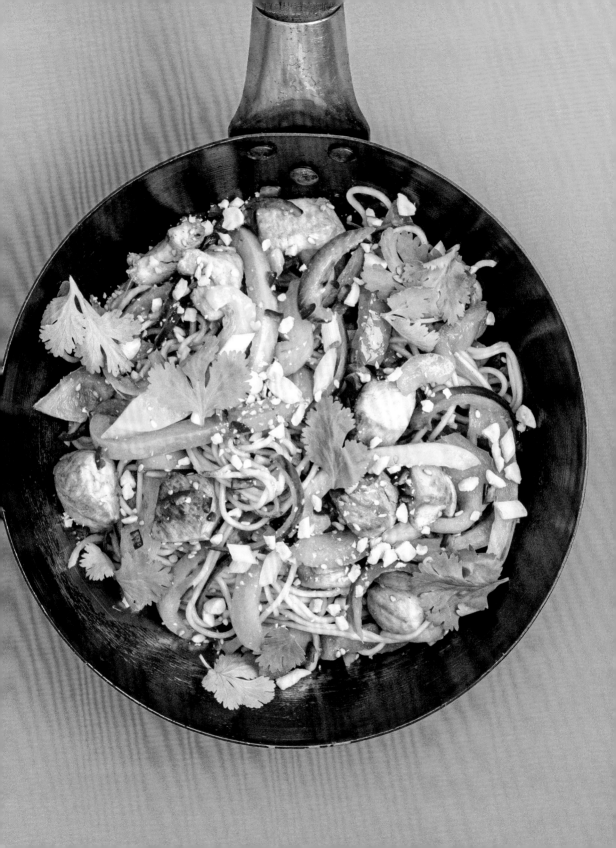

CHICKEN PAD THAI

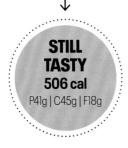

TASTY
744 cal

STILL TASTY
506 cal
P41g | C45g | F18g

This Thai favourite is packed full of flavour. Unfortunately, restaurant versions are usually full of calories, too. But by reducing the sesame oil from 20ml to 5ml and the peanuts from 30g to 10g, you can still enjoy the classic textures and taste of pad Thai while saving 238 calories.

TAKES 15 minutes

50g fresh rice noodles
5ml olive oil
5g brown sugar
150g skinless chicken breast, cut into 4cm pieces
1 tsp garlic powder
50g fresh bean sprouts
2 spring onions, finely sliced
Juice of ½ lime , plus a wedge to serve

10ml light soy sauce
10ml fish sauce
1 red chilli, deseeded and finely chopped
1 medium egg
10g unsalted peanuts, crushed
Small handful of freshly chopped coriander
Black pepper

1. Half-fill a medium saucepan with water and bring to the boil. Add the noodles and simmer for 4–6 minutes until tender. Drain and set aside.
2. While the noodles are cooking, put a medium frying pan over a medium heat, then add the oil, brown sugar, chicken and garlic powder. Cook for 5 minutes.
3. Reduce the heat, then add the bean sprouts, spring onions, lime juice, soy sauce, fish sauce and red chilli, then season with pepper and cook for a further 5 minutes.
4. Crack in the egg and stir thoroughly for 3–4 minutes.
5. Plate up the noodles, followed by the chicken mixture, garnishing with the crushed peanuts, lime wedge and chopped coriander.

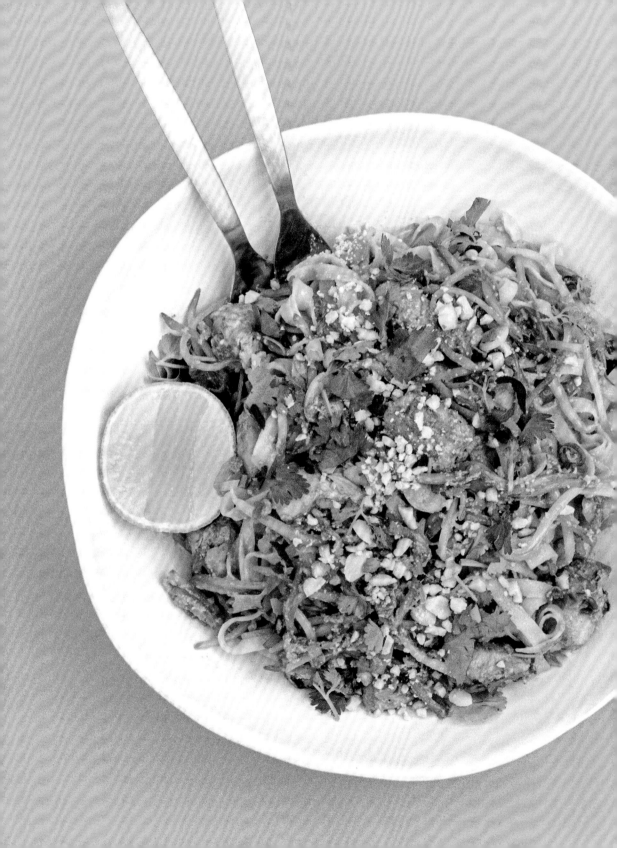

CHINESE-STYLE CHICKEN
& EGG-FRIED RICE

Chinese takeaways and recipes can often be loaded with oil and sugar, which ramp up the calories. This isn't a problem if eaten in moderation, but the calories can add up eventually. By swapping a traditional sauce for one lower in calories, reducing the usual 30ml cooking oil to 10 sprays of oil, plus 5ml of olive oil for the rice, and switching chicken thighs for breast, you can save a huge 335 calories and still enjoy a delicious Chinese-style dinner.

TAKES 20 minutes

10 × sprays olive oil cooking spray
125g skinless chicken breast, cut into 3cm pieces
15ml light soy sauce
½ red pepper, sliced
20g light soft brown sugar
40ml white wine vinegar
1 medium egg

5ml olive oil
125g microwaveable cooked, long-grain white rice
2 spring onions, finely sliced
3g sesame seeds
Small handful of freshly chopped coriander
Black pepper

1. Spray a medium saucepan with the oil and set over a medium heat. Add the chicken and cook for 5 minutes.
2. Reduce the heat, add the soy sauce, red pepper, brown sugar and white wine vinegar. Stir thoroughly until evenly combined and simmer for 6–8 minutes until the sauce has reduced and become slightly sticky.
3. Crack the egg into a small bowl and beat with a fork.

4. Put a small pan over a low heat, add the olive oil, then the cooked rice and stir into the oil with a wooden spoon. Pour in the beaten egg and half the spring onions and cook for 3–4 minutes, stirring continually to coat the rice in the egg mixture.
5. Transfer the egg-fried rice to a serving dish and top with the sticky Chinese chicken. Sprinkle over the sesame seeds, fresh coriander and remaining spring onion, garnish with black pepper and serve.

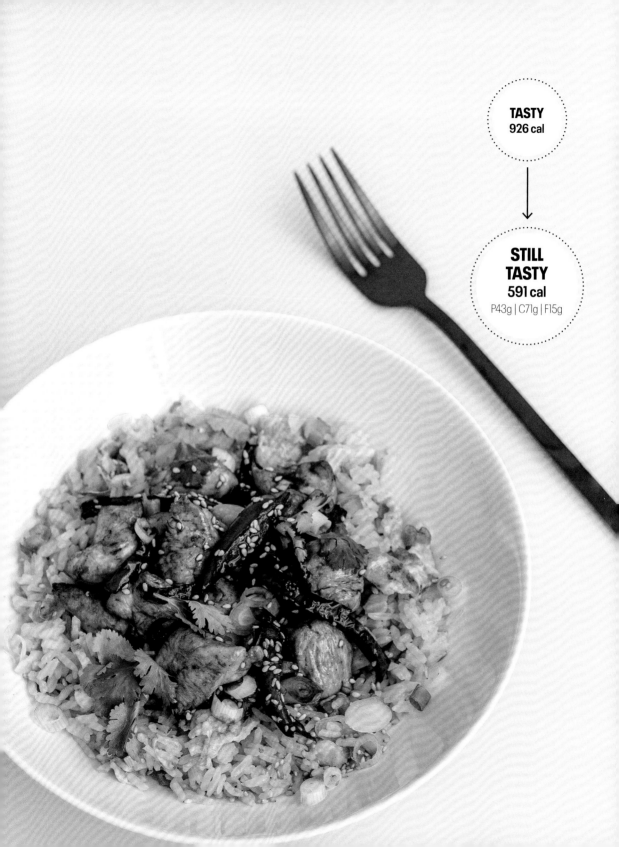

TASTY
926 cal

STILL TASTY
591 cal
P43g | C71g | F15g

BEEF SATAY

TASTY
802 cal

STILL TASTY
626 cal
P55g | C52g | F22g

Satay is a much-loved dish but unfortunately it is often packed full of calories because the sauce contains so much peanut butter and coconut milk. So, if you simply halve the usual 40g peanut butter and swap the coconut milk for skimmed milk, you can save 176 calories and still enjoy those rich satay flavours.

TAKES 15 minutes

125g lean beef, diced into 3cm pieces
5ml olive oil
¼ onion, chopped
10 green beans, halved
125g microwaveable cooked, long-grain white rice
Small handful of freshly chopped coriander
Salt and pepper

For the satay sauce
30g 100% smooth peanut butter
15ml light soy sauce
50ml skimmed milk

1. To make the satay sauce, put the peanut butter, soy sauce and milk in a small bowl and mix with a fork until smooth.
2. Add the diced beef, half the olive oil and some salt and pepper to a separate large bowl and mix with your hands until the beef is completely coated in the oil and seasoning.
3. Put a medium frying pan over a medium heat, then add the remaining olive oil and the onion and green beans. Fry for 2–3 minutes until the onion begins to brown.
4. Add the seasoned beef and fry for 2–3 minutes until sealed. Then reduce the heat and add the satay sauce. Mix with a spatula to coat the beef and vegetables with the sauce and simmer for 5 minutes until the sauce thickens.
5. Microwave the rice on full power for 1½ minutes or cook according to the packet instructions, then transfer to a serving dish. Top with the beef satay and garnish with the coriander and more salt and pepper, if you like.

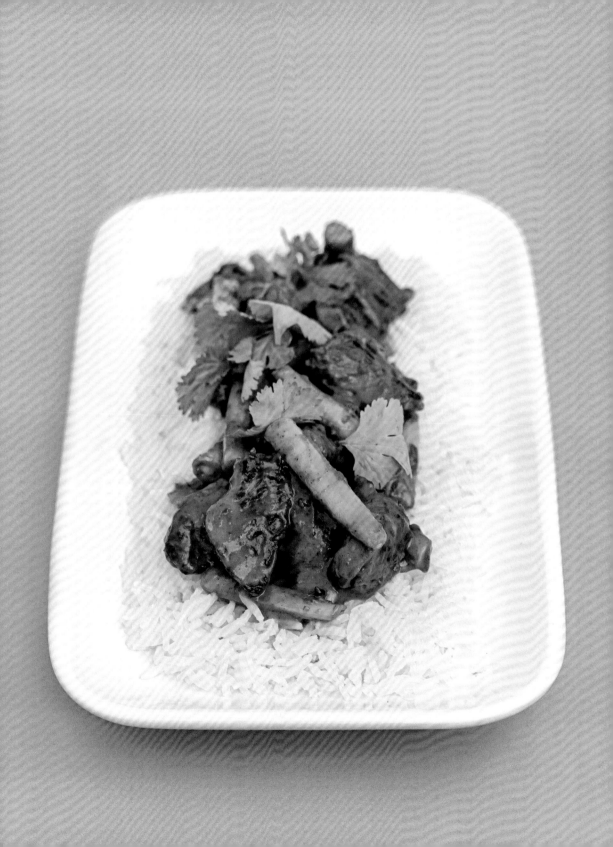

SWEET & SOUR PORK
with rice

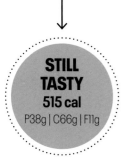

This recipe uses easy ingredient swaps to save you calories. Simply remove the usual 20g sugar and crispy batter. Switch 10ml cooking oil for 10 sprays of oil and leave out the 5ml of oil in the rice. That's a saving of 297 calories. The equivalent to 55g of your favourite chocolate. Or nuts...

TAKES 15 minutes

10 x sprays olive oil cooking spray
125g pork fillet, cut into 4cm pieces
½ onion, sliced
½ red pepper, sliced
50g mangetout
1 tsp ground cinnamon
10ml light soy sauce
1 tsp grated fresh ginger
50ml pineapple juice
30g canned pineapple chunks, drained
50ml cider vinegar
10ml passata
125g microwaveable cooked brown rice
Small handful of freshly chopped coriander
Salt and pepper

1. Spray a medium saucepan with the oil and set over a medium heat. Add the pork and onion and cook for 5 minutes until the pork begins to brown.
2. Add the red pepper, mangetout, cinnamon, soy sauce, ginger, pineapple juice and chunks, vinegar and passata, reduce the heat and cook for a further 6–8 minutes until the sauce thickens and reduces slightly.
3. Put the cooked rice in a small, heatproof bowl and mix with the coriander and some salt and pepper. Microwave on full power for 2 minutes.
4. Transfer the rice to a serving dish, top with the sweet and sour pork and serve.

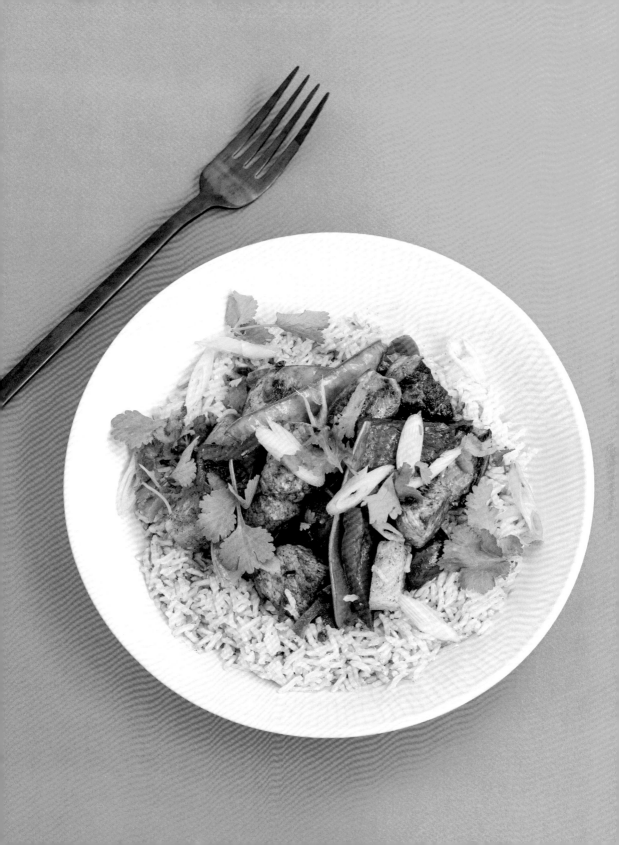

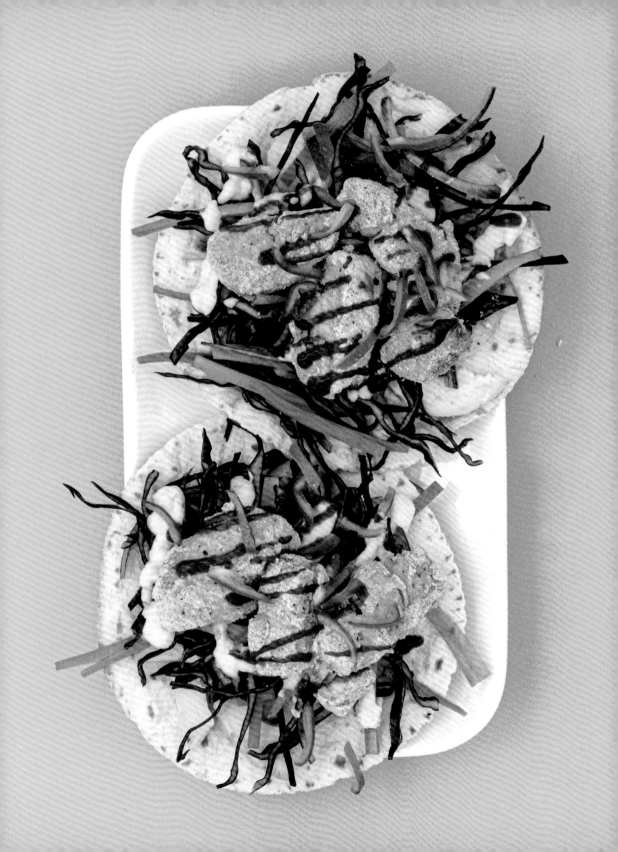

FISH TACOS
with sweetcorn relish

TASTY
922 cal

STILL TASTY
575 cal
P44g | C57g | F19g

This is one of my favourite dishes. Tacos often contain an abundance of sauces and relishes which skyrockets the calorie count. But, as always, there are easy ways to keep the great taste of the original and reduce the calories. All you need to do is swap two ingredients for similar ones: breadcrumbs for polenta and mayonnaise for 0% fat Greek yogurt, and you save a massive 347 calories on a delicious, protein-rich dinner.

TAKES 35 minutes

150g skinless cod or haddock
1 medium egg
40g polenta
1 tsp paprika
1 tsp garlic powder
2 mini tortillas
Salt and pepper

For the slaw
¼ carrot, peeled and grated
30g red cabbage, grated
¼ green pepper, finely sliced
¼ red onion, finely chopped
½ small avocado, sliced
Juice of ¼ lemon, plus extra to serve

For the sweetcorn relish
30g frozen sweetcorn
1 tsp garlic powder
50g 0% fat Greek yogurt
Twist of salt
Squeeze of lime

1. Preheat the oven to 200°C and cut the fish into small fingers.
2. Crack the egg into a medium bowl and whisk with a fork. Add the fish and coat in the beaten egg.
3. Put the polenta, paprika, garlic powder and some black pepper in a separate medium bowl and mix together. Then add the fish pieces, one at a time, coating completely in the polenta. Place the coated fish pieces on a foil-lined baking tray and bake for 20–25 minutes.
4. Meanwhile, add the slaw ingredients to a large bowl and mix thoroughly with your hands. Set aside.
5. To make the sweetcorn relish, put the frozen sweetcorn in a small saucepan, cover with water and set over a high heat. Bring to a simmer and cook for 2 minutes, then drain and rinse in cold running water. Transfer the sweetcorn, yogurt, lime and salt into a blender or food processor and mix together until a chunky texture is achieved.
6. When the fish is cooked, microwave the mini tortillas for 20 seconds to heat. Then divide the cooked fish, slaw and sweetcorn relish evenly between both tortillas. Drizzle more lemon juice over the top and serve.

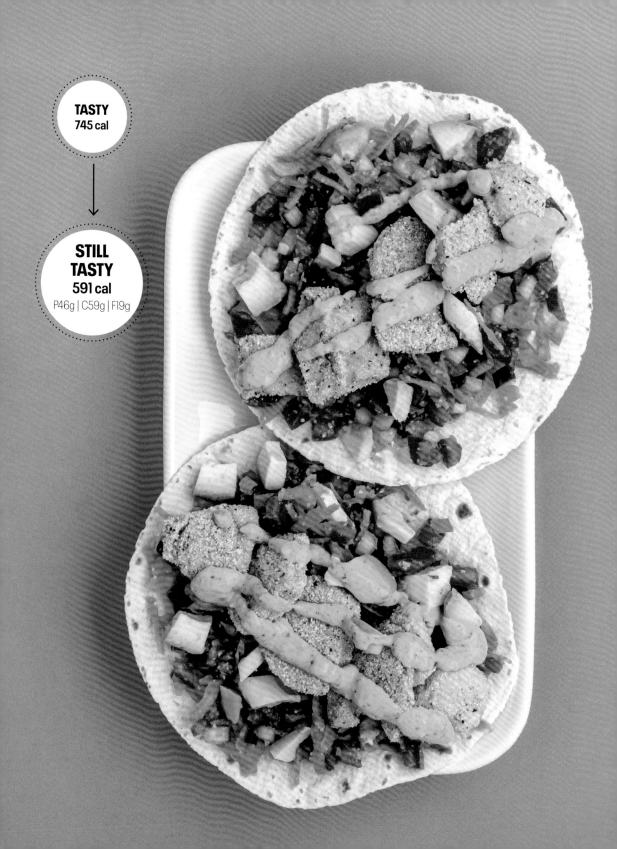

TASTY
745 cal

STILL
TASTY
591 cal
P46g | C59g | F19g

CRISPY CHICKEN TACOS
with salsa & pea relish

This easy taco recipe is a must-try. I've swapped the usual breadcrumb coating on the chicken for polenta and switched the soured cream for 0% fat Greek yogurt to save you 154 calories. Enjoy!

TAKES 30 minutes

1 medium egg
100g skinless chicken breast,
   cut into 3cm pieces
30g polenta
½ tsp salt
1 tsp black pepper
2 mini tortillas

For the salsa
¼ red pepper, finely chopped
2 tomatoes, finely chopped
50g cucumber, finely chopped
¼ carrot, peeled and grated
½ small avocado, finely chopped
Juice of ½ lime
1 tsp garlic powder

For the pea relish
30g frozen peas
50g 0% fat Greek yogurt
Small handful of freshly chopped
   flat-leaf parsley
Squeeze of lemon juice
Twist of salt

1. Preheat the oven to 180°C.
2. Crack the egg into a medium bowl and whisk with a fork. Add the chicken pieces and coat in the beaten egg.
3. Put the polenta, salt and black pepper in a separate small bowl. Coat the chicken pieces in the polenta mixture before transferring to a foil-lined baking dish. Bake for 25 minutes, moving around with tongs halfway through cooking to ensure they are crispy all over.
4. While the chicken is cooking, put all the salsa ingredients in a large bowl and mix thoroughly with your hands. Set aside.
5. Fill a small saucepan one-quarter full of water and add the frozen peas. Set over a high heat and simmer for 2 minutes. Then drain and rinse in cold water to cool. Mash the peas with a fork until mushy, then add the Greek yogurt, lemon juice, parsley and salt and mix thoroughly.
6. Lightly toast the mini tortillas. Then divide the cooked chicken, slaw and pea relish evenly between both tortillas. Serve.

CHICKEN & PICO DE GALLO
BURRITO

The world-famous burrito is a versatile Mexican dish with plenty of protein and nutrients, but given the amount of ingredients packed inside, they are often full of calories too. So, switch up 20ml cooking oil for low-calorie spray oil, change refried beans to black beans and use 50% reduced-fat Cheddar to enjoy the same-sized burrito, but with 273 fewer calories.

TAKES 20 minutes

10 x sprays olive oil cooking spray
100g skinless chicken thighs, cut into 3cm pieces
½ red onion, sliced
30g black beans, drained and rinsed
1 tsp ground cumin
1 tsp smoked paprika
1 tsp garlic powder
30g green pepper, finely chopped
1 large tortilla wrap
50g microwaveable cooked brown rice
15g 0% fat Greek yogurt
¼ small avocado, mashed
15g 50% reduced-fat Cheddar cheese, grated

For the pico de gallo
1 tomato, finely chopped
½ red onion, finely chopped
Small handful of freshly chopped coriander
Juice of ½ lime
½ green chilli, deseeded and finely chopped
Salt and pepper

1. Spray a medium saucepan with the oil and set over a medium heat. Add the chicken and red onion and cook for 5 minutes.
2. Reduce the heat and add the black beans, cumin, smoked paprika, garlic powder and green pepper. Stir into the chicken and cook for 6–8 minutes. Add a drop of water if the mixture is looking a bit dry.

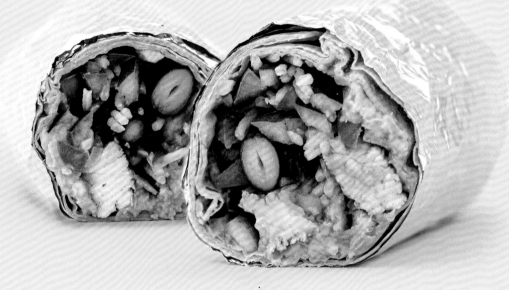

3. To make the pico de gallo, put all the ingredients in a small bowl and mix together with your hands.

4. Put a large pan over a medium heat and warm the tortilla for 30 seconds on each side.

5. Put the cooked rice in a heatproof dish and microwave on full power for 1½ minutes or cook according to the packet instructions, then add to middle of the tortilla with the chicken, veggies and pico de gallo. Top with the Greek yogurt, mashed avocado and grated cheese. Then fold like an envelope and roll. If you're struggling, I recommend finding a video online which shows you the best way to fold your burrito. Enjoy!

BEEF QUESADILLA

This is another popular Mexican dish that's often high in calories. But if you swap 2 tortilla wraps for one, 15ml cooking oil for 5 sprays of oil in a non-stick pan and opt for 50% reduced-fat Cheddar, you can save 364 calories and enjoy the same Mexican flavours.

TAKES 10 minutes

5 x sprays olive oil cooking spray
150g cooked beef, shredded
30g black beans, drained and rinsed
75g passata
1 tsp garlic powder
1 large tortilla wrap
2 tomatoes, chopped

30g mild tomato salsa
Juice of ½ lime
Small handful of freshly chopped
    flat-leaf parsley
30g 50% reduced-fat Cheddar
    cheese, grated

1. Spray a medium saucepan with the oil and set over a medium heat. Add the beef, black beans, passata and garlic powder and cook, stirring, for 1–2 minutes. Remove from the heat.
2. Cut the tortilla in half, then place one half in a large pan over a low-medium heat.
3. Add the beef and black bean mixture, the chopped tomatoes, tomato salsa and lime juice and scatter over the parsley. Lastly, sprinkle over the cheese and place the other tortilla half on top.
4. Increase the heat to medium and cook for 3 minutes until the cheese begins to melt, then carefully flip over with a spatula and cook for a further 3 minutes until both tortilla halves are crispy and golden. Serve.

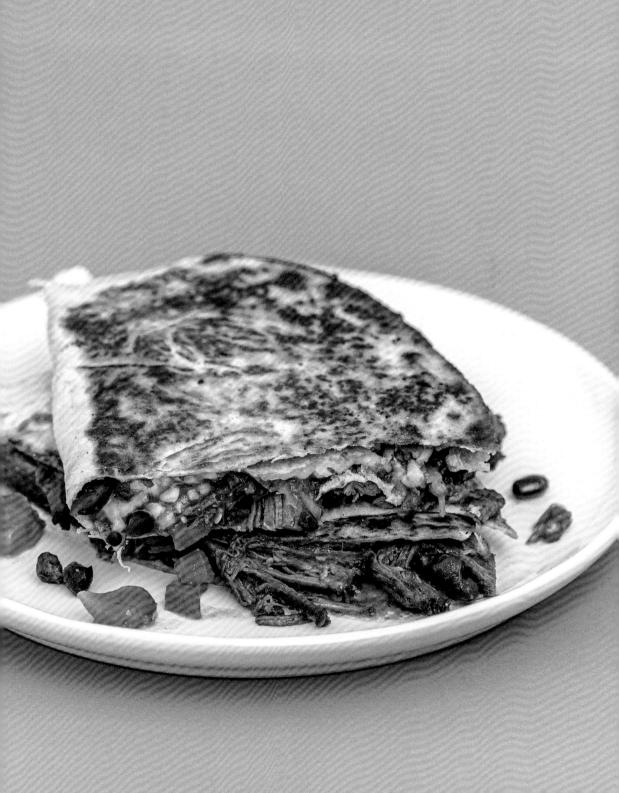

CHICKEN FAJITA

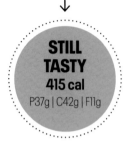

TASTY
521 cal

STILL TASTY
415 cal

P37g | C42g | F11g

Most of the calories in fajitas and other Mexican dishes are found in the sauces and dressings. Here you can save 106 calories and still enjoy a great-tasting fajita by swapping the Cheddar for a 50% reduced-fat version, the soured cream for 0% fat Greek yogurt and halving the usual 10ml olive oil.

TAKES 15 minutes

5ml olive oil	¼ yellow pepper, sliced
1 tsp smoked paprika	¼ small avocado, chopped
100g skinless chicken breast, cut into 3cm pieces	20g 50% reduced-fat Cheddar cheese, grated
50g passata	20g 0% fat Greek yogurt
½ onion, sliced	1 tsp hot sauce
¼ red chilli, deseeded and finely chopped	1 large tortilla wrap
A few baby spinach leaves	Salt and pepper

1. Put a medium saucepan over a medium heat and add the olive oil, smoked paprika and chicken and cook for 5 minutes.
2. Reduce the heat slightly, add the passata, onion and chilli, season with salt and pepper, mix and cook for 6–8 minutes.
3. While the chicken is cooking, arrange the spinach, pepper, avocado, cheese, Greek yogurt and hot sauce in a line in the centre of the wrap.
4. Top with the chicken and tomato mixture, fold, turn over and serve.

SPICY VEGGIE FAJITA

This vegetarian fajita follows the recipe for Chicken Fajita (see opposite) but swaps the chicken for more avocado and black beans. It also ditches the 10ml oil usually used to fry the vegetables and switches Greek yogurt for a 0% fat version. Same great taste with an easy saving of 132 calories.

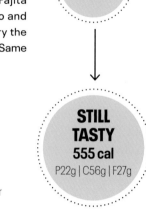

TASTY
687 cal

STILL TASTY
555 cal
P22g | C56g | F27g

TAKES 10 minutes

50g passata
½ onion, sliced
¼ red chilli, deseeded and finely chopped
50g black beans, drained and rinsed
1 tsp smoked paprika
A few baby spinach leaves

¼ red pepper, sliced
1 small avocado, chopped
30g 50% reduced-fat Cheddar cheese, grated
30g 0% fat Greek yogurt
1 tsp hot sauce
1 large tortilla wrap
Salt and pepper

1. Put a medium saucepan over a medium heat, then add the passata, onion, chilli, black beans, smoked paprika, then season with salt and pepper, mix and cook for 6–8 minutes.
2. While the tomato and bean sauce is cooking, arrange the spinach, pepper, avocado, cheese, Greek yogurt and hot sauce in a line in the centre of the wrap.
3. Top with the tomato and bean mixture, fold, turn over and serve.

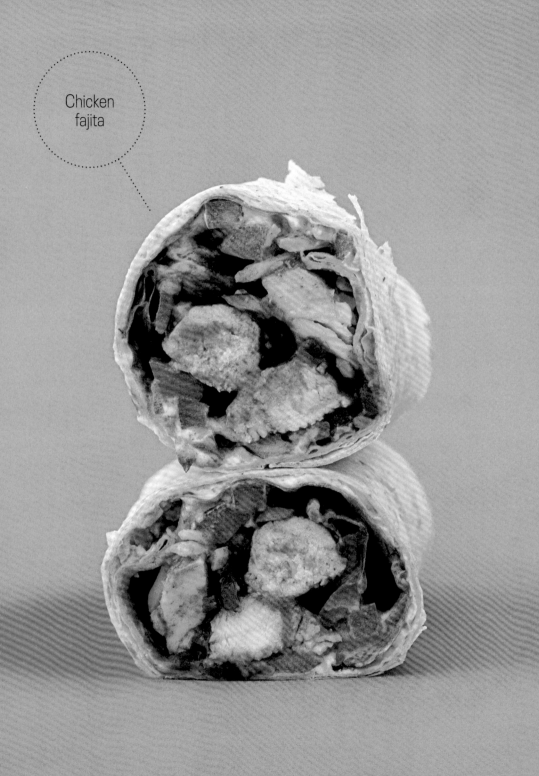

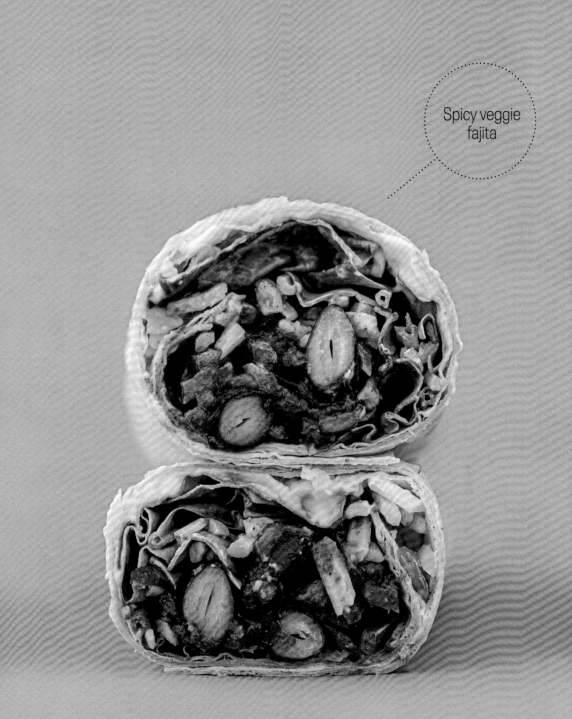

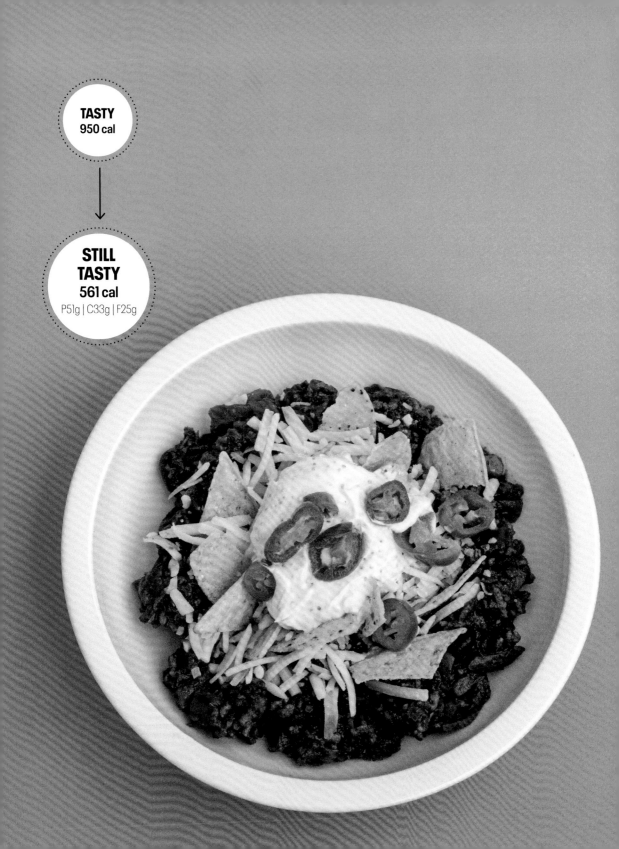

TASTY
950 cal

STILL
TASTY
561 cal
P51g | C33g | F25g

CHILLI BEEF NACHOS

This classic combo is loved by millions around the world. Usually the ingredients make a portion very calorie-dense. But you can still enjoy the same flavours and portion AND lose weight if you simply swap the 20% fat beef mince for 5% fat, American cheese for 50% reduced-fat Cheddar, 15ml cooking oil for 5ml and 100g soured cream for 50g 0% fat Greek yogurt. A huge saving of 389 calories. If you previously treated yourself to nachos once a month, you can now enjoy them far more regularly.

TAKES 15 minutes

For the chilli beef
5ml olive oil
150g 5% fat beef mince
½ onion, chopped
2 garlic cloves, crushed
200ml passata
30g kidney beans, drained and rinsed
½ green pepper, chopped
1 tsp ground cumin
1 green chilli, deseeded and finely chopped
½ tsp mild chilli powder

For the toppings
50g 0% fat Greek yogurt
1 tsp garlic powder
20g tortilla chips
40g 50% reduced-fat Cheddar cheese, grated
1 jalapeño chilli, chopped

1. Put a medium saucepan over a medium heat and add the olive oil, beef mince, onion and garlic. Cook for 3 minutes until the mince starts to brown. Then reduce the heat slightly, add the remaining chilli beef ingredients and simmer for a further 10 minutes, stirring occasionally with a wooden spoon.
2. When the chilli beef is nearly cooked, mix the Greek yogurt and garlic powder together in a small bowl until smooth.
3. Transfer the cooked chilli beef to a serving dish, leaving room to add the tortilla chips.
4. Put the tortilla chips in a heatproof bowl, topwith the cheese and microwave on full power for 30–45 seconds until the cheese has melted. Scatter over the chopped jalapeño and serve alongside the chilli beef.

LAMB MOUSSAKA

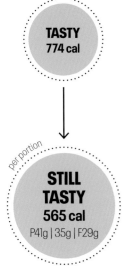

TASTY
774 cal

per portion

STILL TASTY
565 cal
P41g | 35g | F29g

This traditional Greek recipe is the ideal dish for a dinner party or family meal. If you're not feeding a crowd, you can freeze the remaining portions to enjoy at a later date. My version switches 20% fat lamb mince for a low-fat option, changes the 180g crème fraîche to half-fat and Cheddar cheese to a 50% reduced-fat variety for a saving of 209 calories per portion. The best bit is that it still tastes just like the original moussaka recipe!

TAKES 1 hour
MAKES 4 portions

600g potatoes, peeled and finely sliced
1 tbsp garlic purée
2 tsp ground cumin
1 tsp ground cinnamon
1 tsp dried oregano
500g 10% fat lamb mince
10ml olive oil

1 onion, finely chopped
400g passata
2 medium aubergines, peeled and cut into 1cm slices
180g half-fat crème fraîche
100g 50% reduced-fat Cheddar cheese, grated
Salt

1. Preheat the oven to 200°C.
2. Half-fill a large saucepan with water, bring to the boil, then add the finely sliced potatoes. Reduce the heat and simmer for 15 minutes until soft. Drain and rinse in cold water, then leave to cool.
3. While the potatoes are cooking, put the garlic purée, cumin, cinnamon, oregano, lamb mince and a pinch of salt in a large bowl. Mix together with your hands until evenly combined.
4. Put a large pan over a high heat and add half the olive oil followed by the chopped onion and lamb mince. Cook for 3–4 minutes until the mince begins to brown. Then stir in the passata and cook for a further 2 minutes. Remove from the heat.
5. Put a separate large pan over a medium heat and add the remaining oil. Slightly salt the sliced aubergine, then add in batches and cook for 2 minutes on each side until slightly shrunken, lightly golden and tender. Pile the cooked aubergine slices on a side plate while frying the remaining slices.
6. Add a 1cm layer of the lamb to a 25cm square baking dish, followed by a layer of potatoes, then a layer of aubergine.
7. Add the remaining lamb then the remaining aubergine and potato slices.
8. Top with the crème fraîche and spread evenly with a knife, then scatter over the cheese.
9. Bake for 30–35 minutes until golden. Serve.

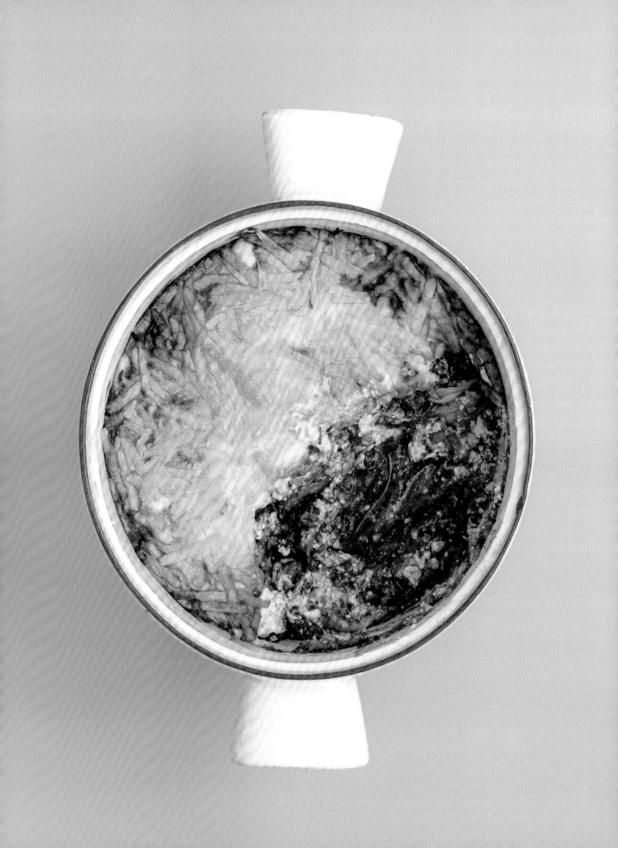

HUNTER'S CHICKEN
& MASH

You might assume that you could never eat a dish including cheese, pancetta and mashed potato and still lose weight. But you're wrong. Reduce the pancetta from 50g to 30g, Cheddar from 40g to 20g (as well as opting for a low-fat variety) and swap the traditional mashed potato packed with 10g butter to a mash made from potato, swede, 2g butter and skimmed milk and you can enjoy all of the same flavours AND save 288 calories.

TAKES 35 minutes

30g smoked pancetta slices
150g skinless chicken breast
100g potato, peeled and cut into 2cm pieces
100g swede, peeled and cut into 2cm pieces

15ml skimmed milk
1 tsp dried coriander
15g barbecue sauce
20g 50% reduced-fat Cheddar cheese, grated
Salt and pepper

1. Preheat the oven to 200°C.
2. Wrap the pancetta slices around the chicken breast, then place on a foil-lined baking tray and cook for 25 minutes.
3. While the chicken is cooking, half-fill a large saucepan with water and bring to the boil. Add the chopped potato and swede and boil for 15–20 minutes until tender. Drain.
4. Mash the cooked vegetables in the saucepan with a potato masher until smooth, then add the milk and dried coriander, season with salt and pepper and mix with a wooden spoon until evenly combined. Keep over a very low heat to stay warm, stirring occasionally.
5. Spread the barbecue sauce over the chicken, followed by the grated cheese. Then return to the oven for a further 5 minutes until the cheese has melted.
6. Serve the chicken alongside the vegetable mash.

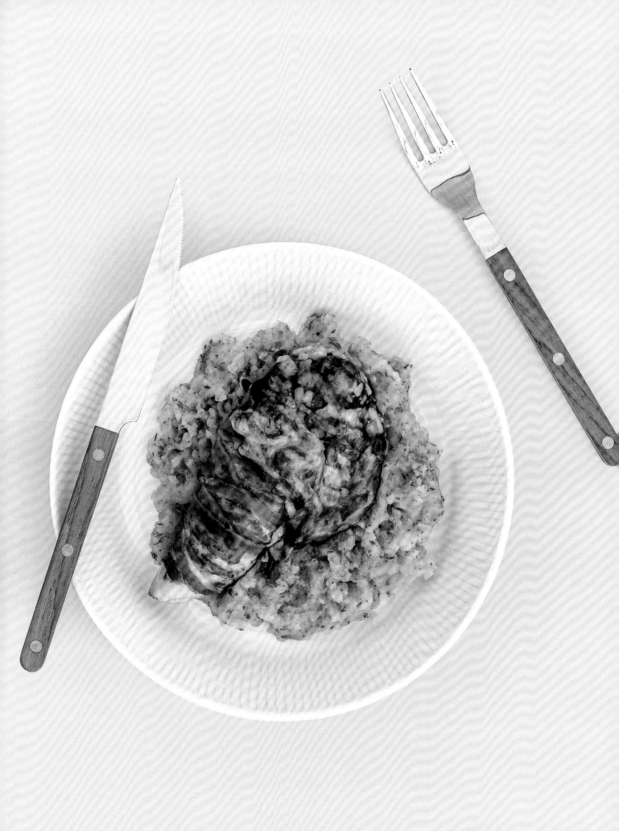

CHICKEN PARMIGIANA

This dish can still taste just as good as the original but with 265 fewer calories by making only a couple of simple adjustments. Swap the usual hefty 60g mozzarella for 40g of a reduced-fat version, then ditch the 15ml cooking oil used to fry the breaded chicken and grill it instead.

TAKES 20 minutes

2 x 100g skinless chicken breasts
1 medium egg
30g dried breadcrumbs
1 tsp garlic powder
1 tsp black pepper
10g Parmesan cheese, grated
250ml passata
½ red onion, roughly chopped
½ red pepper, roughly chopped

20g tomato purée
1 tsp paprika
1 tsp dried basil
40g reduced-fat mozzarella, grated
2 large round lettuce leaves, chopped
5ml balsamic vinegar
3 cherry tomatoes, chopped
Salt

1. Preheat the grill to high.
2. Wrap the chicken breasts in clingfilm, then bash with a rolling pin until they are about 2cm thick.
3. Crack the egg into a large bowl and whisk with a fork until smooth. Put the breadcrumbs in a separate large bowl and mix in the garlic powder, black pepper and grated Parmesan.
4. Dip the chicken in the beaten egg, then in the breadcrumbs mixture until completely coated.
5. Transfer the breaded chicken to a foil-lined baking tray and grill for 5 minutes on each side until crispy.
6. While the chicken is cooking, add the passata, red onion and red pepper to a food processor and blitz until smooth. Then transfer to a small saucepan over a medium heat and add the tomato purée, paprika, basil and a pinch of salt. Simmer for 3–4 minutes until the sauce has reduced and thickened.

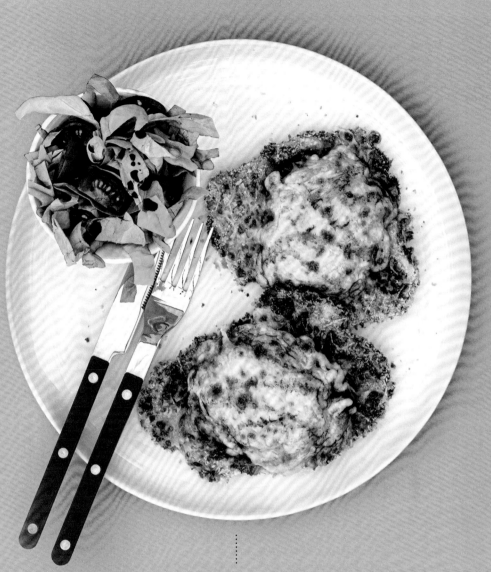

7. Transfer the breaded chicken breasts to the centre of an ovenproof dish and pour the passata sauce over each breast, allowing the sauce to trickle down the sides into the dish.

8. Scatter over the mozzarella and grill for 3–4 minutes until the cheese is melted and turning golden. Remove the chicken onto a serving plate with a spatula.

9. Combine the lettuce, balsamic vinegar and cherry tomatoes and serve alongside the chicken.

THAI RED CURRY

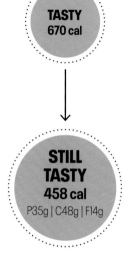

TASTY
670 cal

STILL TASTY
458 cal
P35g | C48g | F14g

You can still enjoy the creamy tastes and mild spices of Thai curries and lose weight. But as with many curries, the sauce and choice of meat makes them calorie-dense. Two simple swaps make all the difference – switch 100ml coconut milk for a light version and 125g chicken thighs for chicken breast and you save 212 calories.

TAKES 15 minutes

5ml sunflower oil
½ red onion, chopped
125g skinless chicken breast, cut into 3cm pieces
2 garlic cloves, crushed
100ml light canned coconut milk
25g red Thai curry paste

½ red pepper, sliced
5 green beans, halved
Juice from ½ lime
½ red chilli, deseeded and chopped
Small handful of freshly chopped coriander
125g microwavable basmati rice

1. Put a medium saucepan over a medium heat and add the sunflower oil, red onion, chicken breast and garlic. Cook for 5 minutes, stirring regularly.
2. Reduce the heat, stir in the coconut milk, curry paste, red pepper, green beans, lime juice, chilli and coriander. Simmer for 7–8 minutes, stirring regularly.
3. Just before serving, microwave the rice on full power for 2 minutes or cook according to the packet instructions. Then transfer the rice to a serving bowl and top with the Thai chicken curry. Serve.

CHICKEN BIRYANI

Swapping the 15g butter or ghee often used in a restaurant biryani for 5g butter and switching chicken thighs for breast saves you 152 calories on this fragrant Indian favourite.

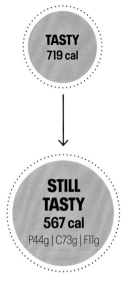

TASTY
719 cal

STILL TASTY
567 cal
P44g | C73g | F11g

TAKES 20 minutes

150g skinless chicken breast, cut into 3cm pieces
1 tsp ground turmeric
1 tsp medium curry powder
1 tsp ground cinnamon
10g salted butter
3 garlic cloves, crushed
1 tsp freshly grated ginger
1 onion, sliced

2 tbsp garam masala
225ml water
200g cooked pilau rice from a packet
Juice of ¼ lemon, plus 2 slices to serve
Small handful of freshly chopped coriander
4 twists of salt

1. Put the chicken, turmeric, curry powder and cinnamon in a large bowl and mix with your hands until the chicken is completely coated in the spices.
2. Put a large saucepan over a medium heat, then add the butter, garlic, ginger and onion. Fry for 2–3 minutes until the onion begins to brown.
3. Stir in the spiced chicken and garam masala and cook for 3 minutes, stirring regularly with a wooden spoon.
4. Then add the water, cooked rice, lemon juice and coriander and stir thoroughly until evenly combined. Reduce the heat, cover the pan with a lid and simmer for 10 minutes, stirring occasionally. Season with salt to taste and serve with the lemon slices on the side.

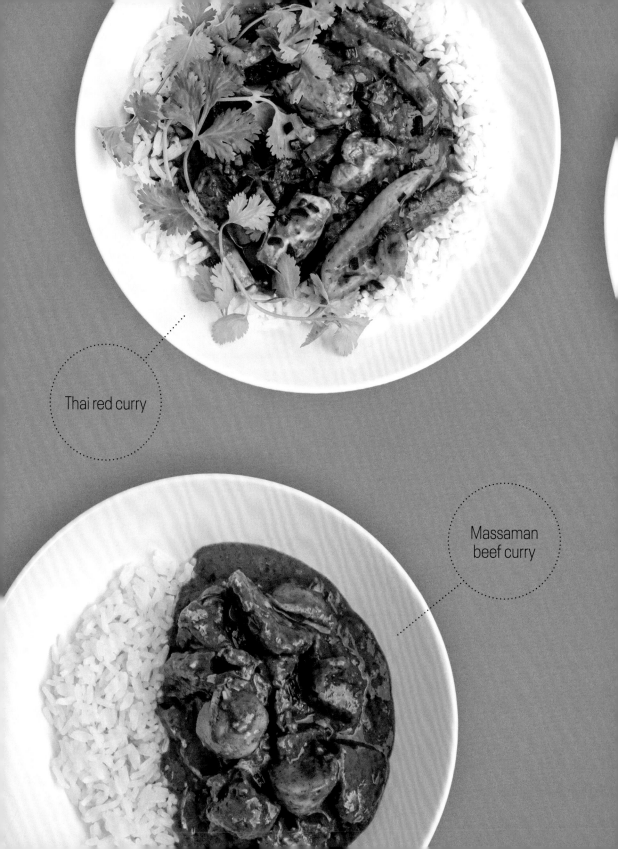

Thai red curry

Massaman
beef curry

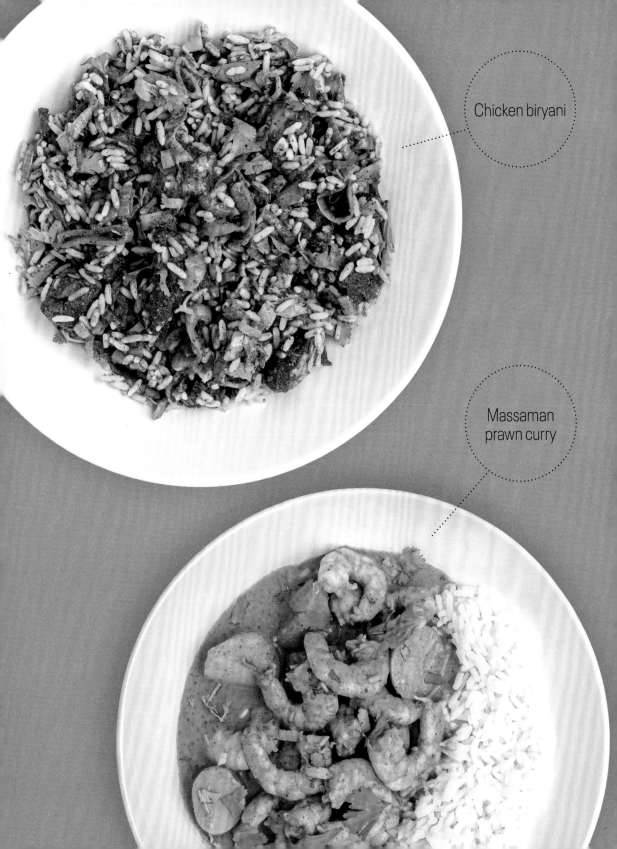

Chicken biryani

Massaman
prawn curry

MASSAMAN
BEEF CURRY

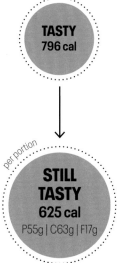

TASTY
796 cal

per portion

STILL
TASTY
625 cal

P55g | C63g | F17g

By switching out the 70g butter usually used to cook the beef for 15g and swapping the coconut milk for a light version, you can save 171 calories while still getting the same rich beef curry.

TAKES 1 hour
MAKES 5 portions

15g unsalted butter
1kg braising beef, cut into 3cm pieces
350ml light coconut milk
40g plain flour
1 beef stock cube
350ml water
400g baby potatoes, scrubbed and chopped into 3cm pieces
125g microwaveable cooked basmati rice per portion
Juice of 1 lime
Large handful of freshly chopped coriander

For the massaman sauce
1 onion, roughly chopped
4 garlic cloves
2 tbsp massaman curry paste
2 red chillies, deseeded and roughly chopped
1 tsp ground cinnamon
1 tbsp ground cumin
1 tsp dried coriander
2 tsp salt
1 tsp black pepper

1. Add all the ingredients for the massaman sauce to a blender or food processor and blitz into a paste.
2. Put a large saucepan over a medium heat and melt the butter. Add the beef and sear for 3–4 minutes, stirring occasionally with a spatula.
3. Reduce the heat and add the massaman sauce to the beef. Cook gently for 2–3 minutes.
4. Add the coconut milk, flour, beef stock cube and water and stir thoroughly, then cover and simmer for 5 minutes.
5. Remove the lid and add the potatoes to the beef, mixing in thoroughly. Place the lid back on and simmer for a further 35 minutes until the potatoes are soft and the beef is tender.
6. When the curry is nearly cooked, microwave the cooked basmati rice on full power for 1½ minutes or cook according to the packet instructions.
7. Add the lime juice and coriander to the curry and give it one final mix, then serve alongside the basmati rice.

MASSAMAN
PRAWN CURRY

Why not try this prawn massaman curry too? By reducing the 70g butter usually used to pan-fry the fish to 15g and swapping the coconut milk for a light version, you can save 171 calories per portion and still enjoy the gently spiced massaman flavours.

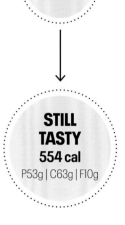

TASTY
725 cal

STILL TASTY
554 cal
P53g | C63g | F10g

TAKES 45 minutes
MAKES 5 portions

15g unsalted butter
1kg uncooked prawns
350ml light coconut milk
40g plain flour
1 vegetable stock cube
5g salt
350ml water
400g baby potatoes, scrubbed and chopped into 3cm pieces
125g microwaveable cooked basmati per portion
Juice of 1 lemon
Large handful of freshly chopped coriander

For the massaman sauce

1 onion, chopped
4 garlic cloves
2 tbsp massaman curry paste
2 red chillies, deseeded and roughly chopped
1 tsp ground cinnamon
1 tbsp ground cumin
1 tsp dried coriander
2 tsp salt
1 tsp black pepper

1. Add all the ingredients for the massaman sauce to a blender or food processor and blitz into a paste.
2. Put a large saucepan over a medium heat and melt the butter. Add the prawns and cook for 2 minutes, stirring occasionally with a spatula.
3. Reduce the heat and add the massaman sauce. Cook gently for 2–3 minutes.
4. Add the coconut milk, flour, vegetable stock cube, salt and water and stir thoroughly, then cover and simmer for 5 minutes.
5. Remove the lid and add the potatoes to the prawns, mixing in thoroughly. Place the lid back on and simmer for a further 20 minutes until the potatoes are soft.
6. When the curry is nearly cooked, microwave the cooked basmati rice on full power for 1½ minutes or cook according to the packet instructions.
7. Add the lemon juice and coriander to the curry and give it one final mix, then serve alongside the basmati rice.

CHICKPEA & LENTIL
MASALA

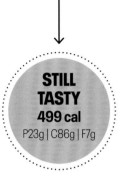

TASTY
778 cal

↓

**STILL
TASTY**
499 cal
P23g | C86g | F7g

As with many curries, cream is usually used to make the sauce in this masala dish. So, switch the 50ml double cream for 50g 0% fat Greek yogurt and swap 10ml cooking oil for 10 sprays of low-calorie spray oil and save yourself 279 calories. Two simple changes for the same delicious veggie masala.

TAKES 20 minutes

10 x sprays butter flavour cooking spray
½ onion, finely chopped
1 tsp ground cumin
1 tbsp tikka masala paste
1 tsp garlic powder
½ vegetable stock cube
200ml cold water
30g split red lentils
75g carrots, peeled and finely chopped

75g canned chickpeas, drained and rinsed
Small handful of spinach
Small handful of freshly chopped coriander
125g microwaveable cooked basmati rice
100g 0% fat Greek yogurt
1 small green chilli, deseeded and finely chopped
Salt

1. Spray a medium saucepan with the oil, set over a medium heat, and add the onion, cumin, masala paste and garlic powder. Stir with a wooden spoon and cook for 3 minutes until the onion begins to brown.
2. Add the vegetable stock cube and water and stir until the cube has dissolved. Then add the lentils, chopped carrot, chickpeas, spinach and coriander. Stir well, reduce the heat, cover and simmer for 20 minutes until the lentils and carrots are tender.
3. Microwave the cooked rice on full power for 2 minutes or cook according to the packet instructions. Then transfer to a serving dish.
4. While the rice is cooking, remove the lid from the pan and mix in the Greek yogurt and green chilli. Cook for 3–4 minutes over a medium heat, then serve with the rice. Season with salt to your taste.

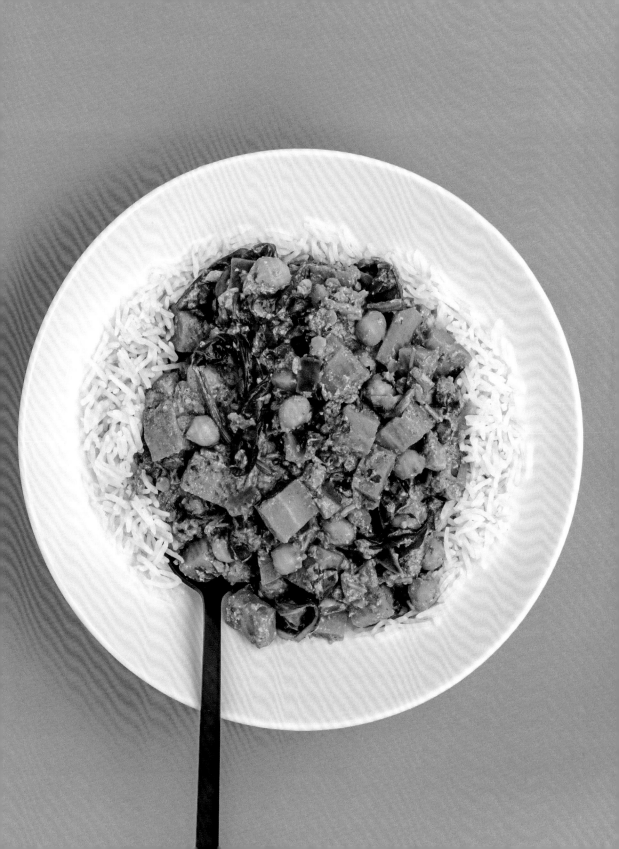

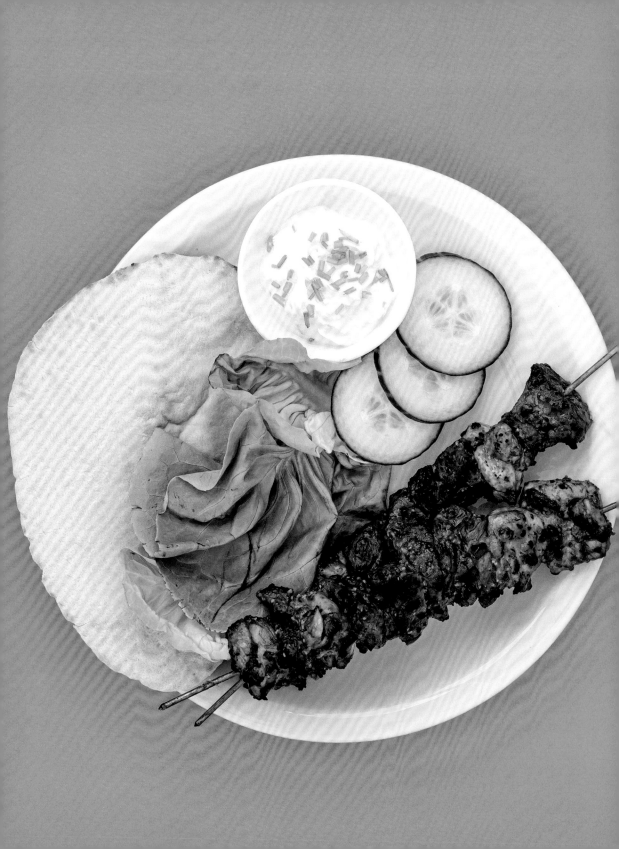

MIXED KEBAB

Most people think they can't eat a kebab and lose or maintain weight, but if a kebab is one of your favourite dishes, then do still eat it, just in moderation. However, if you want to enjoy a kebab more regularly, making a few simple adjustments will reduce the calories significantly. Halve the 20ml olive oil in the marinade, remove the skin from the chicken thigh, swap ribeye steak for fillet and switch 75g Greek yogurt for 50g 0% fat Greek yogurt to keep eating those kebabs, while saving 206 calories with ease.

TAKES 15 minutes

50g lamb steak
50g fillet steak
50g boneless, skinless chicken thigh
1 pitta
1 round lettuce, chopped
20g cucumber, sliced
½ tomato, sliced
50g 0% fat Greek yogurt
½ tsp garlic powder
3 coriander stalks, finely chopped

For the marinade
10ml olive oil
1 tsp smoked paprika
10ml tomato ketchup
5g plain flour
1 tsp garlic powder
Juice of ½ lime
½ red chilli, deseeded and finely chopped (optional)

1. Prepare the marinade by mixing all the ingredients together in a large bowl with a fork until smooth.
2. Chop each piece of meat in half, trying to maintain a rectangular shape, creating 6 pieces of meat (2 of each) in total. Add the meat to the marinade and use your hands to coat it completely. Transfer to a container and marinate in the fridge for 4–6 hours for best results.
3. Preheat the grill to high.
4. Put the meat on to a 20–25cm metal skewer and place on a small, shallow, foil-lined baking tray. Grill for 5 minutes, then rotate the kebab 90 degrees with an oven mitt and grill for a further 5 minutes.
5. While the meat is cooking, slice open the pitta and add the lettuce, cucumber and tomato. Mix the yogurt, garlic powder and coriander together in a small bowl.
6. Remove the meat from the skewer and add to the pitta. Drizzle the yogurt dressing over the top. Serve.

BARBECUE RIBS & MASH

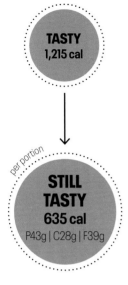

TASTY
1,215 cal

per portion

STILL
TASTY
635 cal

P43g | C28g | F39g

An average portion of restaurant ribs and mash contains around 1,215 calories! This is due to the fat on the meat, the sugar and honey added to the barbecue sauce and the large amounts of butter and cream in the mashed potato. So, by cutting much of the fat off the ribs, ditching the sugar and honey in the barbecue sauce, reducing the amount of butter in the mash and switching the potatoes for sweet potatoes, swede and carrots, you can save a MASSIVE 580 calories and still enjoy an indulgent barbecue-flavoured feast.

PREP 35 minutes
COOK 1 hour 20 minutes
MAKES 4 portions

1kg pork ribs, fat removed
1 tbsp smoked paprika
1 tbsp black pepper
1 tsp salt
1 tsp dried oregano
1 tsp garlic powder
100g barbecue sauce

For the mash
200g sweet potatoes, peeled and chopped into 2cm pieces
500g swede, peeled and chopped into 2cm pieces
200g carrots, peeled and chopped into 2cm pieces
10g unsalted butter
1 tsp salt
Small handful of freshly chopped flat-leaf parsley

1. Put the ribs in a large saucepan and cover them with water. Put the pan over a medium heat and add the smoked paprika, black pepper, salt, dried oregano and garlic powder. Bring to the boil, then reduce the heat and cook gently for 20 minutes.
2. Preheat the oven to 160°C.
3. Remove the ribs from the pan with a pair of tongs and transfer to a 30 x 20cm ovenproof baking dish. Pour the barbecue sauce evenly over ribs, cover with foil and cook for 1 hour 10 minutes–1 hour 20 minutes.

4. While the ribs are cooking, fill a large saucepan with water and put over a medium heat. Add the sweet potatoes, swede and carrots and cook for 20–25 minutes until tender. Drain.

5. Return the vegetables to the pan and mash with a potato masher until smooth. Mix in the butter, salt and parsley.

6. When the ribs are ready, transfer them to a serving dish alongside the vegetable mash and serve.

BBQ PULLED PORK
& APPLE SAUCE BUN

If you like slow-cooked meat, then this is the dish for you. Simply prepare the pork shoulder and leave to slow-cook for 4 hours for a succulent meal packed with protein. Remove the skin from the pork shoulder or buy a skinless cut, make your own apple sauce and swap the brioche bun for a regular white or brown one to save 353 calories while tucking into this deliciously classic pork and apple combo.

TAKES 4 hours
MAKES 5 portions

1 tsp salt	**For the apple sauce**
1 tsp garlic powder	2 apples, peeled and cored
1kg boneless pork shoulder , fat	300ml water
and skin removed	1 tsp ground cinnamon
150g barbecue sauce	Pinch of salt
70g white or brown bun	

1. Preheat the oven to 160°C.
2. Scatter the salt and garlic powder over a large chopping board. Roll the pork shoulder over the seasoning before wrapping it tightly in kitchen foil and placing it on a large, shallow baking tray. Cook for 4 hours.
3. Forty-five minutes before the pork is cooked, start preparing the apple sauce. Chop the apples into 1cm cubes and add to a medium saucepan. Put the pan over a high heat, add the water and bring to the boil, then reduce the heat and simmer for 15–20 minutes. Drain out any water through a sieve, returning the softened apples to the pan. Mash the apples with a potato masher until smooth, then mix in the cinnamon and salt with a wooden spoon.

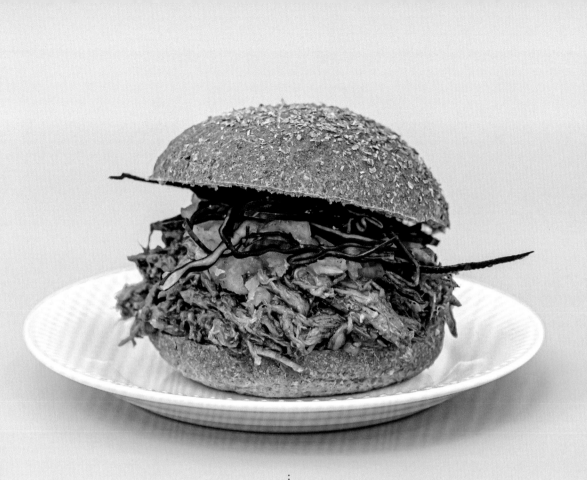

4. Unwrap the pork – it should be falling apart. Use a tablespoon to remove the meat juices to a small bowl, then add the barbecue sauce and mix together with a fork.

5. Tear up the pork with a fork until shredded, cutting off any fatty bits and discarding. Add the barbecue sauce to the shredded pork and mix through.

6. Slice open the bun, add a fifth of the pulled pork and a fifth of the apple sauce. Serve. Store the rest of the pulled pork and apple sauce in separate containers in the fridge or freezer – the pork will keep for 2 days in the fridge and up to 2 months frozen. The apple sauce will last for 2 weeks in the fridge.

CLASSIC BEEFBURGER

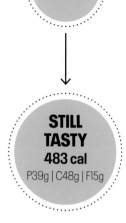

TASTY
684 cal

STILL TASTY
483 cal

P39g | C48g | F15g

Burgers are usually seen as off-limits if you want to lose weight. But this doesn't have to be the case if you understand the ingredients. By just switching 150g 20% fat beef mince for the same quantity of 5% fat mince, you can enjoy the same-sized burger delight, but save 201 calories without even noticing the difference.

TAKES 10 minutes

150g 5% fat beef mince
5ml olive oil
5g plain flour
1 tsp dried basil
½ tsp salt
5 x sprays butter-flavour cooking spray

¼ onion, finely chopped
70g sesame-topped burger bun
10g tomato ketchup
10g tomato relish
2 gherkin slices
1 slice of tomato
Small handful of baby spinach

1. Put the beef mince, olive oil, flour, dried basil and salt in a large bowl and mix thoroughly with your hands. Form the mixture into a large ball, then press into a 2cm-thick burger patty.
2. Spray a small frying pan with the cooking spray, set over a high heat and add the burger patty and onion. Cook the burger for 1 minute on each side to seal the meat. Then reduce the heat to low-medium and cook for a further 3 minutes on each side.
3. Slice open the bun and spread over the ketchup and relish. Then add the cooked burger and onion followed by the gherkin, tomato and spinach. Serve.

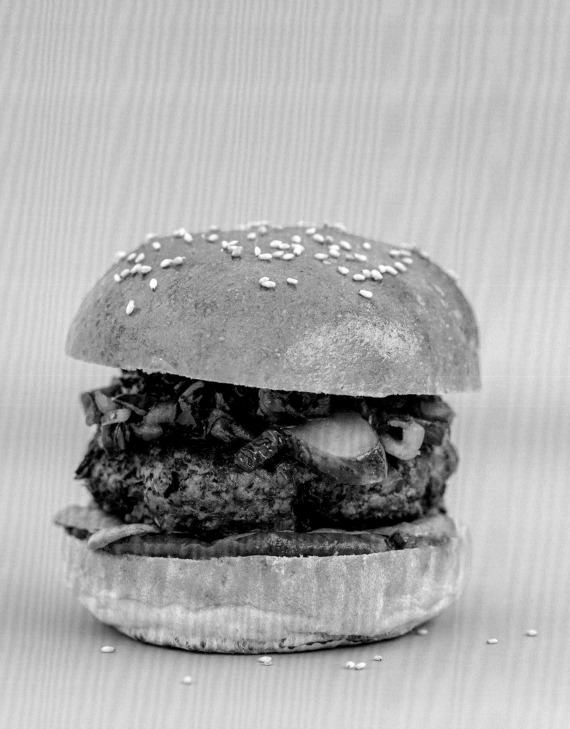

LAMB & MINT BURGER
with garlic dip

If you are presented with a burger and dip your taste buds will probably be salivating only for your conscience to stop you taking that first delicious bite due to the calories they contain. However, altering 30g mayonnaise for 100g 0% fat Greek yogurt and 20% fat lamb mince for a 10% fat version saves 294 calories and you get to enjoy the same great-tasting burger, plus more than three times the amount of garlic dip!

TAKES 20 minutes

150g 10% fat lamb mince
¼ red onion, finely chopped
5g fresh mint, finely chopped
1 garlic clove, crushed
1 tsp dried oregano
1 tsp salt
1 tsp black pepper
10ml olive oil
Small iceberg lettuce leaf
3 slices of cucumber
1 tomato slice
10g red onion, sliced

For the garlic dip
100g 0% fat Greek yogurt
1 tsp garlic powder
Twist of salt and pepper
Small handful of finely chopped chives
70g white or brown roll

1. Put the lamb mince, red onion, mint, garlic, dried oregano, salt, black pepper and half the olive oil in a large bowl and mix thoroughly with your hands. Form the mixture into a firm ball before pressing into a burger patty around 3cm thick.
2. Put a small frying pan over a medium heat then add the remaining olive oil followed by the lamb patty. Cook for 2 minutes on each sides to seal the meat, then reduce the heat to low and cook for a further 5 minutes on each side until the burger becomes slightly charred.
3. While the burger is cooking, prepare the garlic dip by mixing the Greek yogurt, garlic powder, salt, pepper and chives together in a small bowl.
4. Slice open the roll, add the lettuce, cucumber, tomato and red onion, then the lamb burger and a quarter of the garlic dip, saving the remainder for dipping with each bite.

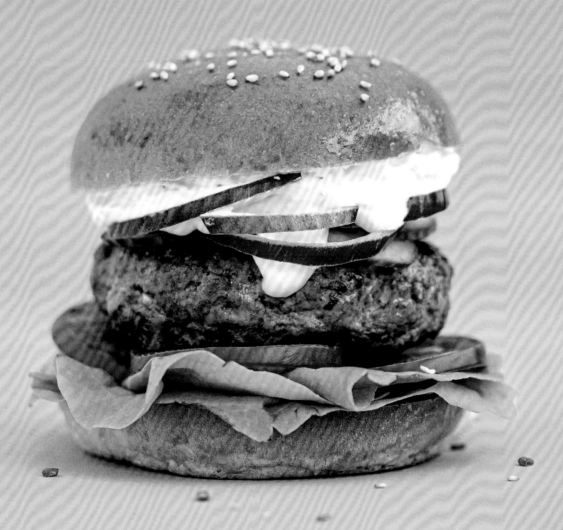

BUFFALO CHICKEN BURGER
with rainbow slaw

This is another of my favourite recipes. By halving the usual 30g butter in the buffalo sauce, switching the natural yogurt to a 0% fat version, ditching 15ml cooking oil for 15 sprays of low-calorie cooking oil and opting for a light mayo, you can enjoy the rich flavours and textures of this breaded burger, but save 225 calories to support your calorie deficit, too.

The buffalo sauce makes 15 portions, so any leftovers can be stored in an airtight container in the fridge for 3 weeks. As for the rainbow slaw, you can also store the remaining portions in a container in the fridge for up to 5 days. You can also use the slaw in the Veggie Burger on page 197.

TAKES 20 minutes

125g skinless chicken breast
20g panko breadcrumbs
1 tsp garlic powder
1 medium egg
10g plain flour
15 x sprays olive oil cooking spray
70g wholemeal roll

For the buffalo sauce
(Makes 15 portions)
100ml hot pepper sauce
100g 0% fat natural yogurt
15g unsalted butter
1 tsp Worcestershire sauce
1 tsp garlic powder
1 tsp paprika
½ tsp salt

For the rainbow slaw
(Makes 5 portions)
½ small red cabbage, grated
1 small carrot, peeled and grated
½ red onion, sliced
1 tsp cider vinegar
40g light mayonnaise

1. To make the buffalo sauce, add all the ingredients to a small saucepan over a low heat and simmer for 4–5 minutes, stirring occasionally. Remove from the heat, and transfer to a clean serving bottle or jar. Chill in the fridge.
2. Preheat the grill to high.
3. Wrap the chicken breast in clingfilm and bash with a rolling pin until it is 2cm thick.

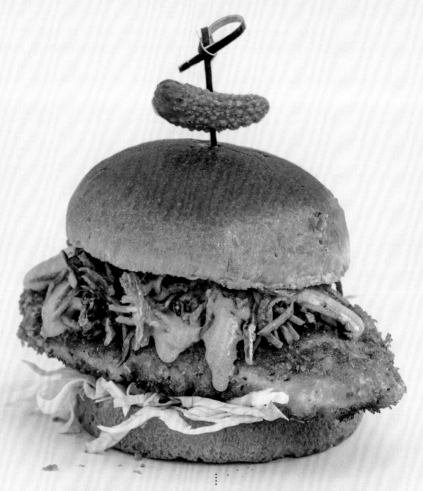

4. Mix the breadcrumbs and garlic powder together in a large bowl. Crack the egg into a separate large bowl and beat with a fork until smooth. Add the flour to a third bowl. Cover the chicken breast in the flour, then dip in the beaten egg and finally coat in the breadcrumbs.

5. Spray a medium saucepan with the oil and set over a medium-high heat. Add the breaded chicken and cook for 1 minute on each side until crispy. Transfer to a foil-lined baking tray and grill for 7–8 minutes on each side.

6. While the chicken is cooking, put all the ingredients for the rainbow slaw in a large bowl and mix together with wooden spoon. Transfer to a container and refrigerate until needed.

7. Slice open the roll, add the breaded chicken and a portion of buffalo sauce and rainbow slaw and serve.

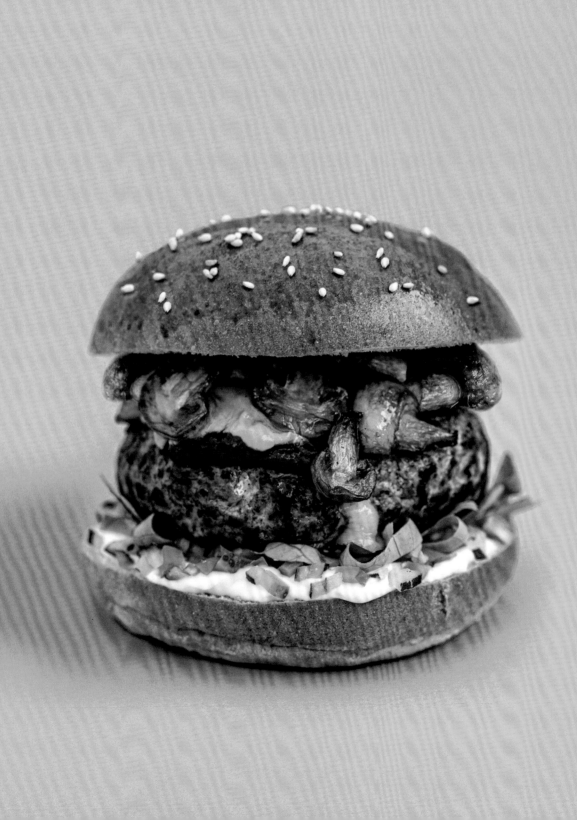

CHEESE-LOADED
BURGER

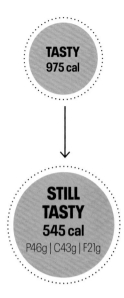

TASTY
975 cal

STILL TASTY
545 cal
P46g | C43g | F21g

Yes, you can stuff cheese in a burger, load up on toppings and still lose weight! Swap the 20% fat pork mince for a 5% fat option, 20ml cooking oil for 20 sprays of low-calorie cooking spray, the Cheddar for a 50% reduced-fat version and the mayonnaise for a light variety to save a massive 430 calories while tucking into a juicy, cheese-stuffed burger with all the toppings. Enjoy this one in all its glory...

TAKES 15 minutes

150g 5% fat pork mince
5g plain flour
1 tsp paprika
½ tsp salt
½ tsp black pepper
½ tsp garlic powder
1 tbsp peeled, grated apple
5ml olive oil
25g piece of 50% reduced-fat Cheddar cheese, 1cm thick

20 x sprays olive oil cooking spray
4 button mushrooms, chopped
¼ onion, finely chopped
70g white roll
5g American mustard
5g light mayonnaise
2 gherkin slices
5g tomato ketchup
Large leaf of round lettuce

1. Put the pork mince, flour, paprika, salt, black pepper, garlic powder, grated apple and olive oil in a large bowl and mix thoroughly with your hands. Form the mixture into a large meatball, then squash the block of cheese into the centre. Flatten into a burger patty, ensuring the cheese is completely covered in the meat.
2. Spray a large frying pan with the oil, set over a high heat and carefully add the patty. Seal for 1 minute on each side, then reduce the heat to medium and cook for 6–7 minutes on each side until slightly charred.

Take care when flipping it over with a spatula to ensure the cheese doesn't spill out.
3. When the burger is halfway through cooking, add the mushrooms and onion to the pan and fry for 5–6 minutes until slightly browned.
4. Slice open the roll, add the cooked burger, then spread over the mustard, top with the onions and mushrooms, then the mayonnaise, gherkins, ketchup and lettuce. Cut in half and serve.

CHEESEBURGER & FRIES

Some fast-food chains offer relatively low-calorie cheeseburgers, but the portion size is usually very small, too. Most larger restaurant versions with extravagant toppings can be calorie-dense – mostly due to the fat content of the ingredients. But by switching 20% fat beef mince for 5% fat, swapping deep-fried fries for oven-baked ones, normal Cheddar for 50% reduced-fat and 10ml cooking oil for 10 sprays of low-calorie spray oil, you can still indulge in a burger, toppings AND fries, but save almost HALF the calories! If you enjoy this once a week for a year, that's a saving of just over 30,000 calories! Or the equivalent of 136 chocolate bars...

TAKES 40 minutes

125g 5% fat beef mince
½ tsp salt
½ tsp black pepper
1 tsp dried oregano
20 x sprays olive oil cooking spray
30g 50% reduced-fat Cheddar cheese, grated or sliced
70g white or brown roll
Small piece of iceberg lettuce
1 slice of tomato
5g tomato ketchup

For the fries
150g potatoes, skin on
5ml olive oil
1 tsp dried Italian herbs
10g tomato ketchup
Salt and pepper

1. Preheat the oven to 200°C.
2. Chop the potatoes into thick-cut fries, then add to a large bowl with the olive oil and dried Italian herbs and some salt and pepper. Mix with your hands until the fries are completely covered in oil and seasoning. Transfer to a baking tray lined with greaseproof paper and cook for 30–35 minutes until golden and crispy.
3. After 20 minutes, put the beef mince, salt, pepper, oregano and 10 sprays of oil in a large bowl and mix together with your hands until completely combined. Form the mixture into a 7–8cm burger patty.

4. Spray a small frying pan with the remaining oil, set over a high heat and add the patty. Sear for 1 minute on each side, then reduce the heat to medium and cook for 4 minutes. Then flip the patty over with a spatula, top with the cheese and cook for a further 4 minutes.
5. Transfer the fries to a serving plate.
6. Slice open the roll, add the cheeseburger, lettuce, tomato and ketchup and serve with the fries and the remaining ketchup on the side.

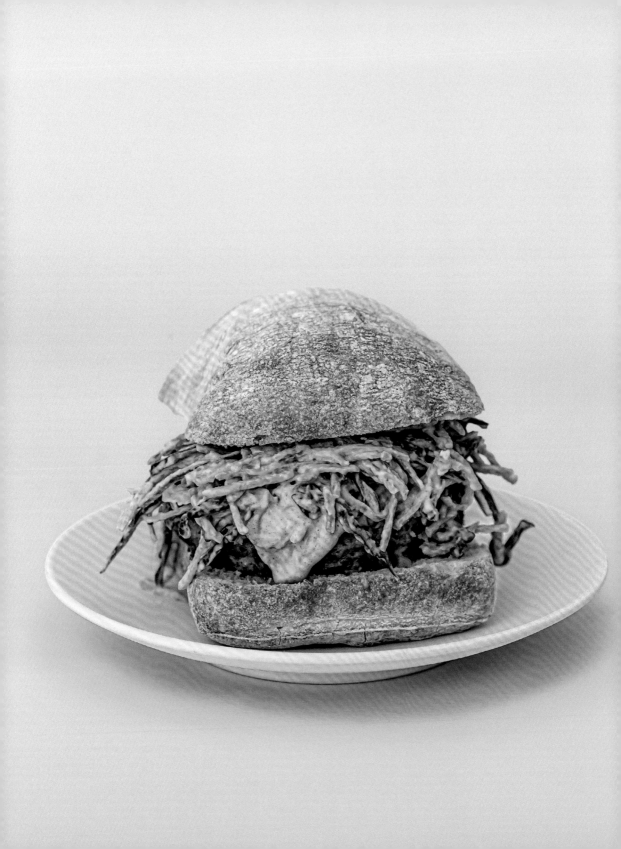

VEGGIE BURGER
with rainbow slaw

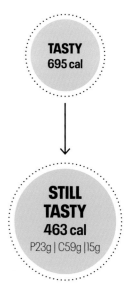

TASTY
695 cal

STILL TASTY
463 cal
P23g | C59g | 15g

People always assume vegetarian burgers are lower in calories than their meat counterparts. While they are more nutrient-dense, you can still save on calories. Just swap 15ml olive oil for 15 sprays of low-calorie cooking oil and switch the mayo for a lighter version and you'll save 232 calories per portion without losing any of the taste.

TAKES 20 minutes

75g button mushrooms, finely chopped
5ml olive oil
50g butter beans, drained and rinsed
50g chickpeas, drained and rinsed
10g dried breadcrumbs
2 garlic cloves, crushed

1 tsp dried oregano
1 tsp garlic powder
15 x sprays olive oil cooking spray
80g ciabatta roll
30g cucumber, sliced
5g Dijon mustard
1 portion of Rainbow Slaw (see page 190)
Salt and pepper

1. Half-fill a small saucepan with water and bring to the boil. Add the mushrooms and cook for 5 minutes until soft. Drain.
2. Transfer the drained mushrooms to a large bowl, add the oil, butter beans, chickpeas, breadcrumbs, garlic, oregano and garlic powder and season with salt and pepper. Mash together with a potato masher until you have a thick paste. Form the mixture into a 2cm-thick burger patty using your hands.
3. Spray a medium frying pan with the oil and set over a medium-high heat. Add the veggie patty and fry for 1 minute on each side, then reduce the heat to low-medium and fry for a further 4 minutes on each side.
4. Slice the ciabatta roll in half and lightly toast. Then add the veggie burger, sliced cucumber, mustard and a portion of rainbow slaw.

CREAMY CHICKEN
& MUSHROOM PIE

People often ban pies when they're trying to lose weight, but recipe names don't mean anything, it's ingredients and their quantities that are important. So, you CAN eat pie! Simply reduce the calories in your version by swapping the chicken thighs for breast, 20ml cooking oil for 20 sprays of oil spray and whole milk for skimmed to save 136 calories per portion.

TAKES 55 minutes
MAKES 4 portions

20 x sprays butter-flavour cooking spray
600g skinless chicken breast, cut into 4cm pieces
2 garlic cloves, crushed
1 red onion, chopped
200g button mushrooms, sliced
40g cornflour, plus extra for dusting (optional)
1 chicken stock cube
250ml water
150ml skimmed milk
Small handful of freshly chopped chives
375g fresh, ready-rolled puff pastry sheet
Salt and pepper

1. Preheat the oven to 200°C.
2. Spray a large saucepan with the cooking spray, set over a medium heat and add the chicken, garlic and onion. Cook for 5 minutes, stirring regularly, until the ingredients begin to brown.
3. Add the mushrooms and cornflour, then stir before adding the chicken stock cube and water, beating with a fork. Stir again, then add the milk and stir until evenly combined. Simmer for 10–15 minutes until the sauce thickens then stir in the chives.
4. Transfer to a 25cm square ovenproof baking dish.
5. Lay the sheet of pastry over the baking dish. If it isn't big enough, scatter 5g of cornflour over a clean surface and roll out the pastry sheet until large enough to fit over the dish. Pinch the pastry to the edges of the baking dish with a fork and trim any overhanging pastry. Cut a hole in the middle for the steam to escape.
6. Bake for 30–35 minutes until the pastry has risen and is golden. Serve.

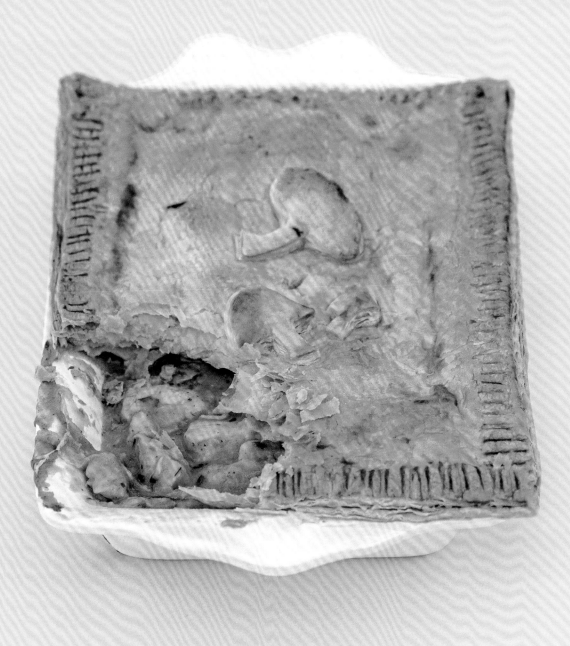

DESSERTS

Many so-called 'healthier' desserts miss the point. The reason you enjoy desserts is because of the sweet ingredients they contain. So, there will be no banning sugar or cream here. In fact, most of the dessert ingredients I've used are in the original recipe.

Instead, I've found ways to reduce the calorie content by adjusting the quantities of calorie-dense ingredients, ensuring that the size of each dessert stays the same, and that the taste is just as sweet and delicious.

NO-BAKE MINI
STRAWBERRY CHEESECAKES

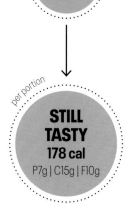

TASTY
352 cal

per portion

STILL TASTY
178 cal

P7g | C15g | F10g

Many people will ban any dessert with the name 'cheesecake' because they are usually so calorie-dense that they are bound to destroy your calorie deficit. However, if you love cheesecake, then eat it. But if you want to enjoy it regularly, making a few simple swaps and adjusting the quantities of some ingredients means you get the same delicious dessert for significantly fewer calories. This recipe switches the traditional full-fat soft cheese and single cream used to make the cheesecake topping for 300g Quark to halve the calories.

PREP 35 minutes
REFRIGERATE 2 hours
MAKES 10 mini cheesecakes

100g cashew nuts, soaked in water for 20 minutes, drained
40g coconut oil
80g soft pitted dates
80g oat bran

20g caster sugar
300g Quark
1 tbsp vanilla extract
Zest and juice of ½ lemon
150g strawberries, hulled and sliced

1. Place the cashew nuts in a bowl of water, soak for 20 minutes, then drain. Next, put the coconut oil in a small, heatproof bowl and microwave on full power for 30 seconds until melted.
2. Put the coconut oil, dates, oat bran and cashews in a blender and blitz until a sticky ball forms. Remove from the blender and press down with damp fingers into 10 × 8–10cm serving dishes until 2cm thick. Refrigerate for 30 minutes.
3. Put the sugar, Quark, vanilla extract, lemon zest and juice in a large bowl and mix until evenly combined.
4. With a spatula, carefully add the topping to the 10 bases and refrigerate for 2 hours to firm up.
5. When you are ready to serve, top the cheesecakes with the sliced strawberries and enjoy.

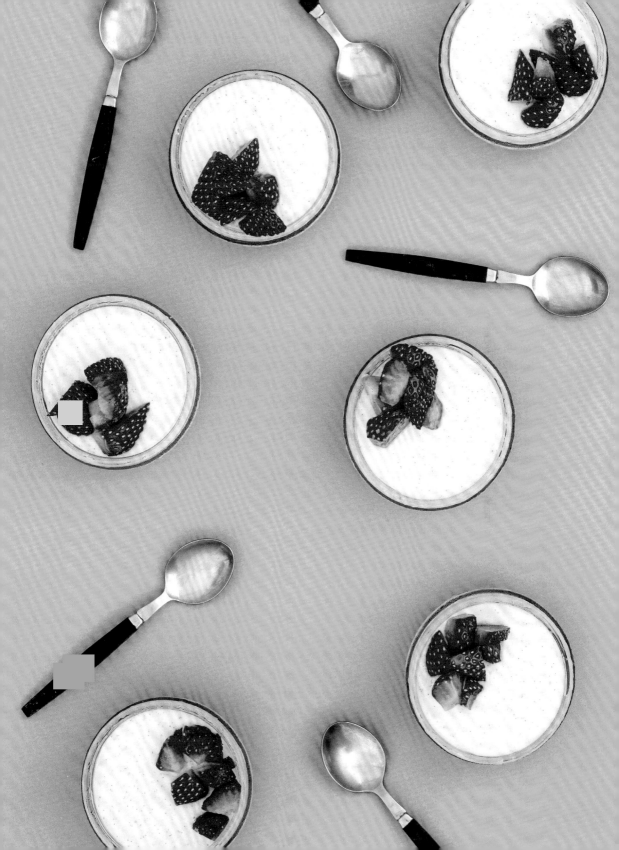

NEW YORK
CHEESECAKE

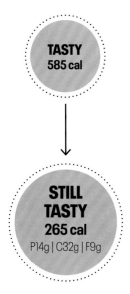

TASTY
585 cal

STILL
TASTY
265 cal

P14g | C32g | F9g

My version of this much-loved American classic ditches the butter and flour, reduces the sugar, switches full-fat soft cheese for a smaller quantity of Quark and uses lemon zest and juice to give the sour flavours you usually get from the soured cream. Simple swaps for a saving of 320 calories.

PREP 45 minutes
COOL 2 hours
CHILL 6 hours or overnight
MAKES 8 portions

10g of coconut oil
20 × sprays butter flavour cooking spray
5 ginger biscuits
5 digestive biscuits
3 medium eggs
500g Quark

200g 0% fat vanilla yogurt
1 tbsp vanilla extract
50g caster sugar
Zest and juice of 1 lemon
25g plain flour
10g dark chocolate, finely grated

1. Preheat the oven to 200°C and line a 20–25cm springform cake tin with baking paper.
2. Add the coconut oil to a small bowl and microwave for 30 seconds to melt. Then add to a blender or food processor with crumbled biscuits and blitz until powdered. Transfer to the base of the cake tin, pressing down with damp fingers so it's evenly distributed.
3. Bake for 5–6 minutes until the base is firm. Remove from the oven and increase the oven temperature to 220°C. Grease the sides of the baking tin with the spray oil using a piece of kitchen paper.
4. Crack the eggs into a large bowl and add the soft cheese, vanilla yogurt, vanilla extract, sugar, lemon zest and juice, and whisk until thoroughly combined.
5. Spread the topping over the biscuit base and bake for 10–12 minutes.
6. Reduce the heat to 110°C and cook for a further 25 minutes until shaking the tin produces slight wobble in the middle of the cheesecake.
7. Turn the oven off and leave the cheesecake inside to cool for 2 hours. Then transfer to the fridge to chill overnight.
8. To serve, loosen the edges with a cake spatula, pull the cake tin lever and release the edges of the tin, leaving the base to serve from. Evenly distribute the grated dark chocolate over the cheesecake. Serve.

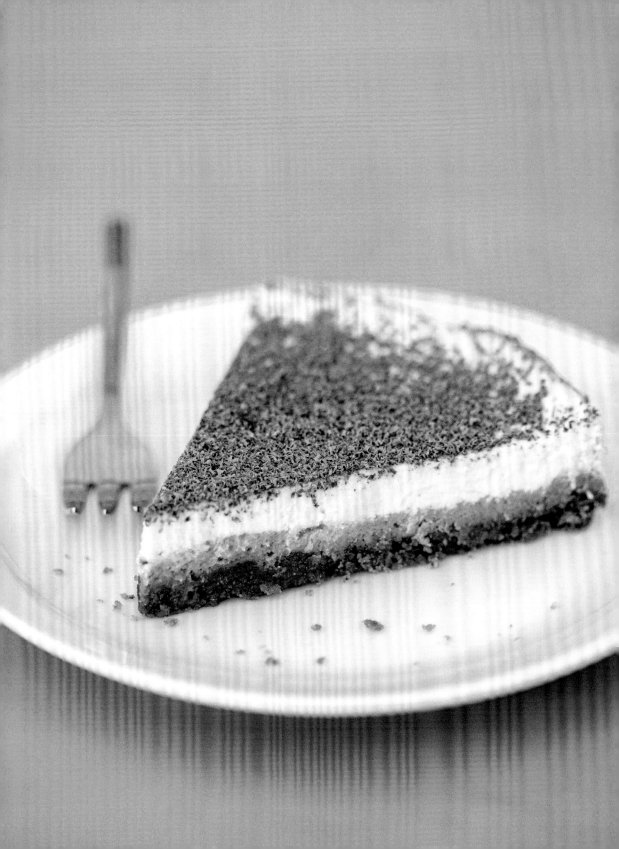

CHOCOLATE & RASPBERRY
MOUSSE

per portion

Simply swap 8 eggs for 8 egg whites, 100ml double cream for 100g 0% fat Greek yogurt and drop the usual 50g sugar and you can save 136 calories every time you enjoy a creamy, chocolatey mousse.

PREP 10 minutes
CHILL 4–5 hours or overnight
MAKES 8 portions

200g milk or dark chocolate   8 medium egg whites
100g 0% fat Greek yogurt   160g raspberries

1. Break the chocolate into a large, heatproof bowl and set over a saucepan half-filled with boiling water. Stir with a wooden spoon until the chocolate has melted. Remove the bowl from the saucepan and leave to cool for 3 minutes before folding in the Greek yogurt with a spatula until evenly combined.
2. Add the egg whites to a separate large bowl and whisk with an electric hand-whisk until stiff.
3. Gradually add the stiff egg whites to the chocolate mixture, folding them in with a spatula until evenly mixed. Divide the mousse evenly between 8 × 8–10cm dishes or ramekins.
4. Refrigerate for 4–5 hours and serve with fresh raspberries.

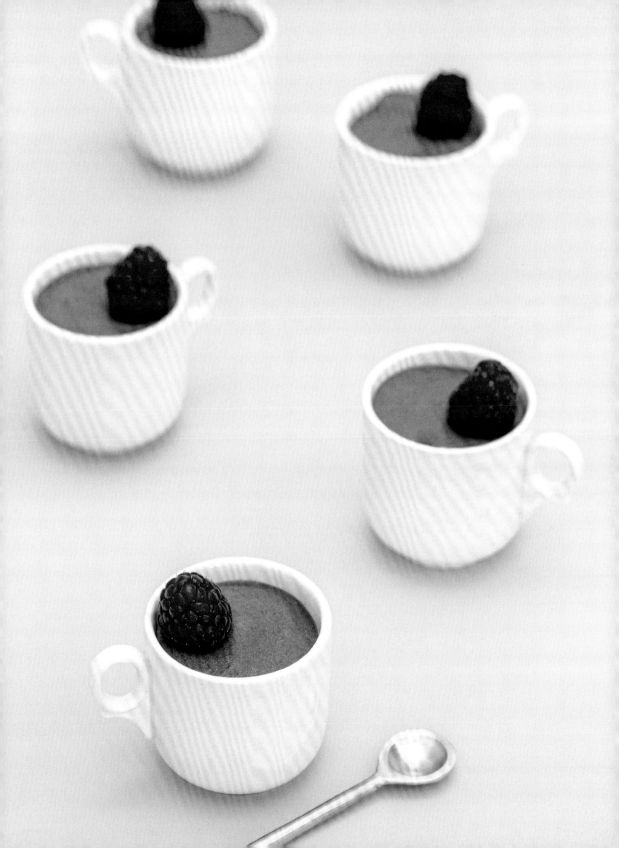

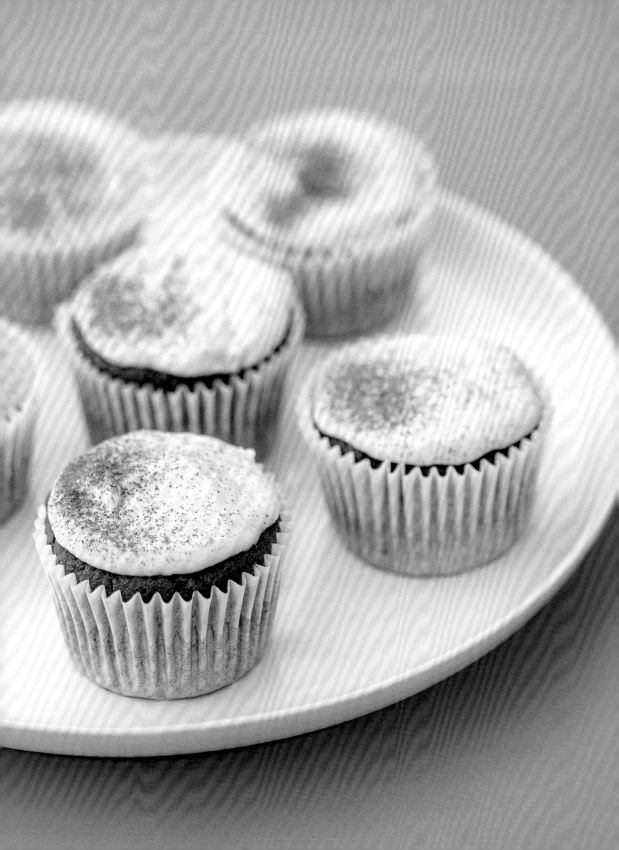

VANILLA CREAM
CARROT CAKES

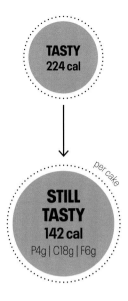

TASTY
224 cal

per cake

STILL
TASTY
142 cal

P4g | C18g | F6g

By reducing the amount of sugar and butter in this recipe, you can keep the unique, sweet flavours of carrot cake while still saving 82 calories.

TAKES 50 minutes
MAKES 10 cakes

10 × sprays olive oil cooking spray
2 small carrots, grated
2 medium eggs
50g self-raising flour
1 tsp bicarbonate of soda
1 tbsp ground cinnamon
30ml maple syrup
10g brown sugar
30g pitted dates
2 tsp vanilla extract

For the cream topping
100g cashew nuts, soaked in water
for 20 minutes
2 tsp vanilla extract
30ml maple syrup

1. Preheat the oven to 190°C.
2. Spray the oil into 10 holes of a 12-hole muffin tray and wipe with kitchen paper.
3. Put all the cake ingredients in a food processor and blend until smooth.
4. Fill each cake holder with a cupcake case, then half-fill each case with batter and bake for 15–20 minutes until risen and golden. Leave to cool for 10 minutes.
5. Drain the cashews and add to a food processor with the vanilla extract and maple syrup. Blend until smooth. You may need to add a drop of water to loosen the mixture a little.
6. Transfer to the fridge to chill for 10 minutes before adding a heaped tablespoon on top of each carrot cake. Then serve or store in an airtight container for up to 5 days.

TIRAMISU

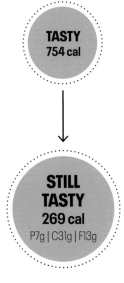

TASTY
754 cal

STILL TASTY
269 cal
P7g | C31g | F13g

If you usually choose tiramisu when eating out, go for it, but bear in mind that an average portion contains around 754 calories due to the amount of mascarpone cheese and double cream. But reduce the mascarpone (and swap it for a light version), switch the double cream for semi-skimmed milk and whipping cream and you can save a massive 485 calories AND still enjoy a delicious tiramisu treat.

PREP 20 mins
CHILL 3 hours
MAKES 6 portions

50g light mascarpone
250g light cream cheese
150g whipping cream
50ml semi-skimmed milk
50g caster sugar
2 tsp vanilla extract

20ml rum or brandy
300ml brewed coffee,
  cooled for 10 minutes
20 ladyfinger biscuits
30g cocoa powder

1. Put the mascarpone and cream cheese in a large bowl and mix with a wooden spoon until evenly combined. Gradually stir in the whipping cream, milk, sugar, vanilla extract and rum or brandy.
2. Pour the cooled coffee into a shallow bowl, then dip one-third of the ladyfingers in the coffee briefly, then use them to line the base of a deep 20cm serving dish.
3. Pour one-third of the cream mixture over the ladyfingers and then sprinkle over 10g of the cocoa powder.
4. Repeat until you have used all the biscuits and the cream layer is on top – you should have 3 layers of each. Use the remaining 10g of the cocoa powder to dust over the top.
5. Refrigerate for 3 hours and then serve.

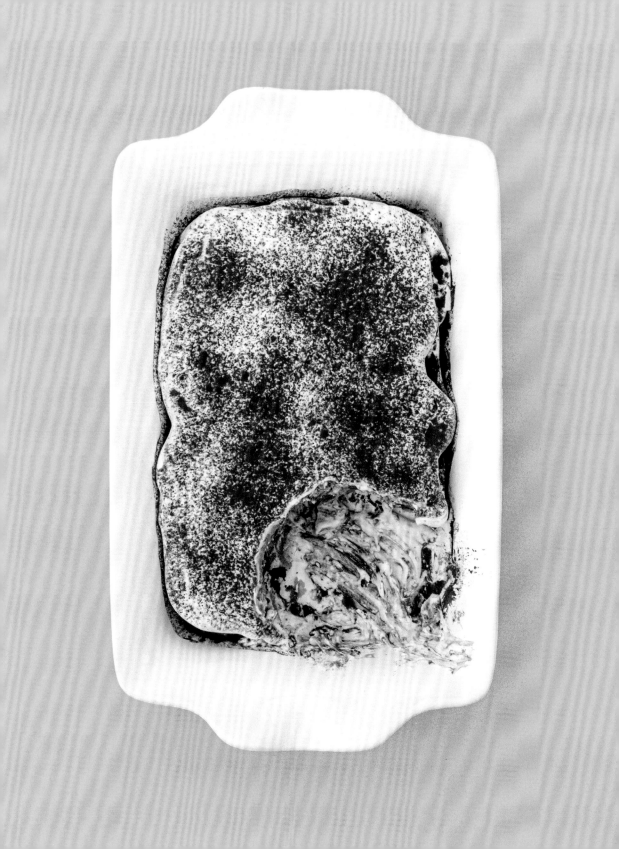

STICKY TOFFEE PUDDING

Sticky toffee pudding is one of the most popular desserts. If you search online to find a lower-calorie alternative they often don't match up to the original in taste. That's why I've included sugar, cream and butter in my recipe, but in smaller quantities, along with some maple syrup. So, you can still enjoy a classic-tasting sticky toffee pudding, but also save 450 calories, allowing you more of your favourite dessert!

TAKES 30 minutes
MAKES 10 portions

10 × sprays butter-flavour cooking spray
75g self-raising flour
1 tsp baking powder
2 medium eggs
15g unsalted butter, softened
20g muscovado sugar
80g pitted dates, soaked in water for 10 minutes
1 tsp vanilla extract
25g black treacle
15g maple syrup

For the toffee sauce
15g muscovado sugar
10g unsalted butter
5g black treacle
20ml single cream
40ml semi-skimmed milk

Serve with
15ml single cream

1. Preheat the oven to 180°C and spray a medium 22cm round cake tin with the oil and smear all over the base and sides with kitchen paper until completely coated. Line with baking paper.
2. Put the self-raising flour and baking powder in a medium bowl and mix together with your hands.
3. Crack the eggs into a separate medium bowl and whisk until smooth. Add the butter and sugar gradually, mixing hard with a wooden spoon before slowly adding the dry ingredients. Mix thoroughly until you have a slightly lumpy batter.

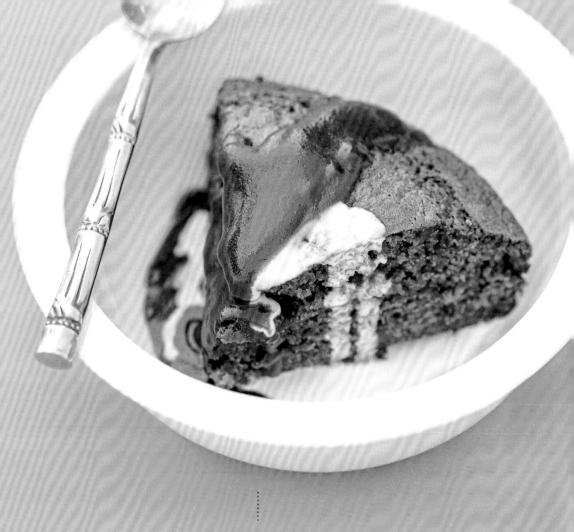

4. Finely chop the soaked dates, add to a food processor and blitz until you have a purée. Add 50g date purée to the batter with the vanilla extract, treacle and maple syrup, stirring to form a lumpy batter.
5. Transfer the batter to the cake tin and bake for 20 minutes until risen.
6. While pudding is baking, make the toffee sauce. Put the remaining 30g date purée, sugar, butter, treacle, cream and milk in a small saucepan and heat gently for 2–3 minutes, stirring constantly until you have a thick sauce.
7. Slice the pudding into 5 portions using a cake knife and pour toffee sauce and single cream over each individual portion.

FRUIT PAVLOVA

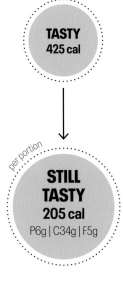

Many reduced-calorie versions of this famous dessert replace sugar with granulated sweetener. Well, not here! You can simply cut the calories by swapping the traditional 500ml double cream for 400g 0% fat Greek yogurt and 100ml whipping cream to maintain the creamy textures. So, save yourself 220 calories and you can enjoy this tasty dessert more regularly...

PREP 15 minutes
BAKE 1 hour
COOL 1½ hours
MAKES 8 portions

4 medium egg whites (160g)
115g caster sugar
115g icing sugar
400g 0% fat Greek yogurt
100ml whipping cream

100g raspberries, halved
100g strawberries, hulled and chopped
1 medium kiwi, peeled and chopped
2 passion fruit

1. Preheat the oven to 120°C and line a baking sheet with grease-proof paper or a silicone mat.
2. Put the egg whites in a clean (metal or glass) mixing bowl, then beat with a hand mixer until they form stiff peaks. Increase the speed and add the caster sugar, 1 tablespoon at a time, leaving a few moments between each spoonful so it's fully combined and doesn't separate later. Once the mixture is thick and glossy, sift in a third of the icing sugar and use a spatula to fold it in. Repeat with the remaining two-thirds. The mix should look smooth and billowy.
3. Use a spoon to dollop the meringue onto the prepared baking sheet. Cook for 1 hour, then leave the door open for a few minutes to let the temperature cool down, then cook for a further 1½ hours. Remove from the oven and leave to cool.
4. Put the Greek yogurt and whipping cream in a large bowl and mix thoroughly with a wooden spoon. Scoop over the pavlova and then scatter with the chopped fruit. Drizzle the passion fruit over the top and serve.

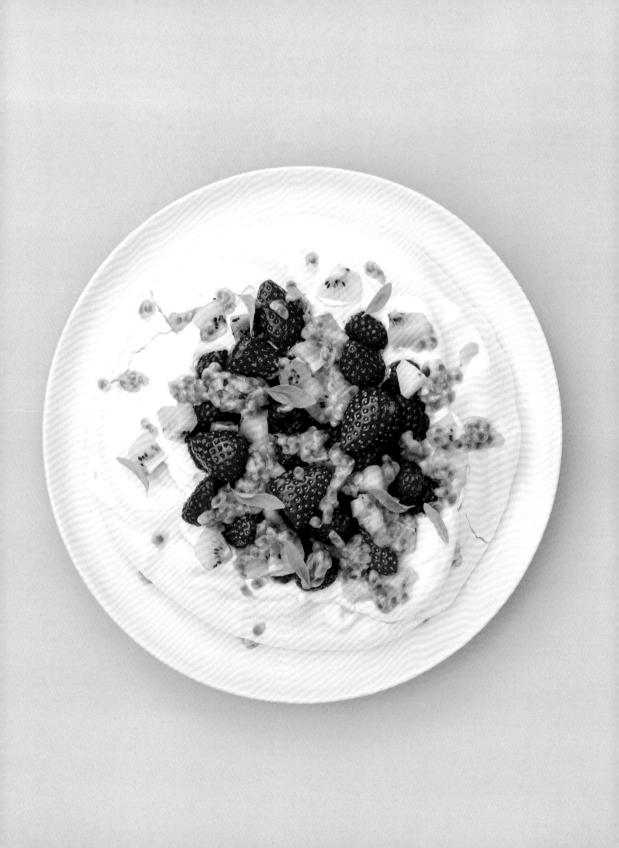

NO-BAKE
BANOFFEE DESSERT

Banoffee pie can be one of the most calorie-dense desserts, largely due to the amount of double cream and toffee. My version swaps 350ml double cream for 250g 0% fat Greek yogurt and 100ml whipping cream and uses light condensed milk to give you the familiar banoffee flavours, but with 257 fewer calories and none of the hassle of baking.

PREP 15 minutes
CHILL 1 hour
MAKES 8 mini desserts

10g coconut oil
120g digestive biscuits (8 biscuits), crumbled
20g butter
20g brown sugar
200ml light condensed milk
50g half-fat crème fraîche
10g cornflour

For the toppings
2 large, ripe bananas
100ml whipping cream
1 tsp vanilla extract
250g 0% fat Greek yogurt
½ tsp instant coffee
10g cocoa powder

1. Put the coconut oil in a small, heatproof dish and microwave on full power for 30 seconds until melted. Then add to a food processor with the digestive biscuits and blitz until you have a moist powder. Divide 20g between 8 × deep 8–10cm round serving dishes.
2. Put the butter and brown sugar in a saucepan over a medium heat and stir until the butter has melted and you have a paste. Gradually add the condensed milk and cornflour and stir until it begins to thicken. Remove from the heat and stir in the crème fraîche. Leave the toffee to cool for 5 minutes to thicken.
3. Split the toffee mixture between 8 serving dishes and chill for 45 minutes–1 hour until set.
4. Cut the bananas into 1cm slices. Distribute half of the slices across the serving dishes on top of the set toffee.
5. Put the whipping cream, vanilla extract and Greek yogurt in a large bowl and mix thoroughly with a wooden spoon until smooth. Divide evenly between the 8 serving dishes, placing on top of the banana.
6. Put the instant coffee in a small bowl and use the end of a rolling pin (or pestle and mortar) to grind into a powder. Add the cocoa powder and mix thoroughly with a teaspoon. Scatter the remaining banana slices evenly over the top of the banoffee desserts, followed by a sprinkling of the coffee/cocoa mixture. Serve.

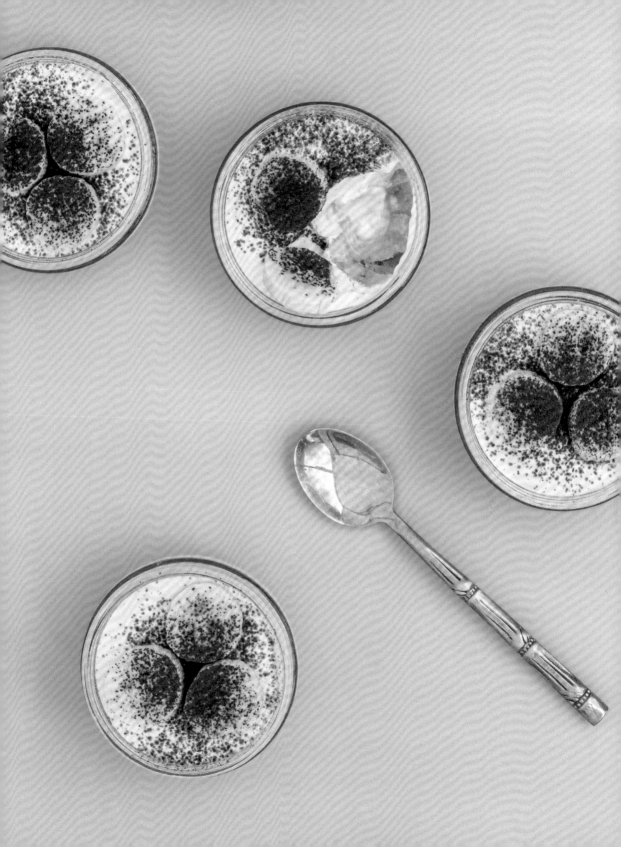

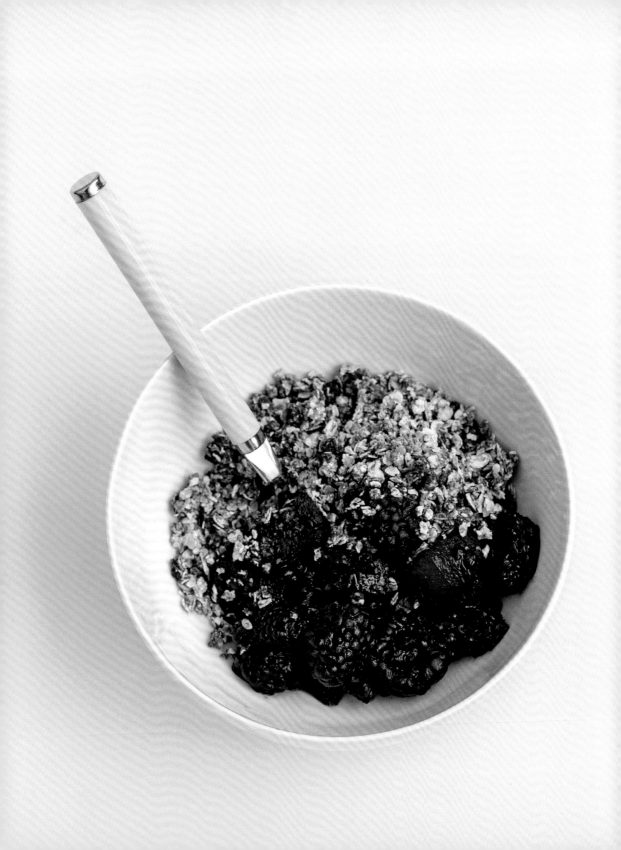

APPLE & BERRY
CRUMBLE

You can significantly reduce the calories in this comforting crumble by simply ditching the usual 100g butter in the topping and swapping the 120g sugar for 75g honey.

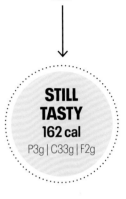

TASTY
347 cal

**STILL
TASTY
162 cal**
P3g | C33g | F2g

PREP 10 minutes
BAKE 30 minutes
MAKES 6 portions

3 medium apples, peeled, cored and finely chopped
100g raspberries
100g blackberries
150g rolled oats

75g runny honey
1 tbsp ground cinnamon
10 sprays of butter-flavour oil spray
5g brown sugar

1. Preheat the oven to 220°C.
2. Add the chopped apples and water to a small saucepan over a medium heat and stew for 10 minutes until soft and tender.
3. Scatter the apples and berries evenly over the base of a large, deep baking dish.
4. Put the oats, honey and cinnamon in a large bowl and mix with a wooden spoon until evenly combined.
5. Scatter the topping over the apples and berries, then evenly spray with spray oil and bake for 30 minutes until the topping is golden and crispy and the apples and berries are tender. Serve with sugar sprinkled on top.

INDEX

ACKNOWLEDGEMENTS

I'd like to thank you for spending your money on my book. I'm delighted and grateful. I hope it empowers you to know that you don't have to ban any foods from your diet to succeed.

Thank you to Ebury and Penguin for having faith in me for a second book and allowing me to help even more people. Thanks to Sophie Yamamoto for her highly skilled book design, and to Hannah Pemberton who shot the brilliant food images throughout the book.

I'd like to thank Jen, my excellent agent who continues to provide outstanding support.

I'd also like to thank my close and extended family for supporting me over the last few years. Without this support I would not be in the position I'm in today.

1

Ebury Press, an imprint of Ebury Publishing
20 Vauxhall Bridge Road
London SW1V 2SA

Ebury Press is part of the Penguin Random House group of companies
whose addresses can be found at global.penguinrandomhouse.com

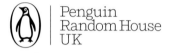

Text © Graeme Tomlinson
Photography by Hannah Pemberton © Ebury Press
Additional photo credits: pages 4, 5, 10, 11, 12 © Graeme Tomlinson

Graeme Tomlinson has asserted his right to be identified as the
author of this Work in accordance with the Copyright, Designs
and Patents Act 1988

This edition published by Ebury Press in 2021
www.penguin.co.uk

A CIP catalogue record for this book is available
from the British Library

ISBN 9781529108354

Designed by maru studio
Colour origination by Altaimage, London
Printed and bound in China by C&C Offset Printing Co., Ltd

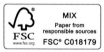

Penguin Random House is committed to a sustainable
future for our business, our readers and our planet. This book
is made from Forest Stewardship Council® certified paper.